Compassion Focused Therapy for Beginners

A Practical Introduction to CFT for Overcoming Shame, Self-Criticism, and Emotional Distress

A guided introduction to the modern compassion-focused tradition, written in plain English for readers without clinical training.

Landry Jerome Humphrey

The content of this book is provided for general informational and educational purposes only. It is not intended as a substitute for professional medical, psychological, psychiatric, or therapeutic advice, diagnosis, or treatment. Always seek the guidance of a qualified mental health professional regarding any concerns about your emotional, psychological, or physical wellbeing. The practices described in this book are not appropriate for every reader or every circumstance, and readers with significant trauma histories, current mental health conditions, or suicidal ideation are strongly encouraged to work with a trained clinician.

All names, characters, scenarios, and case examples presented in this book are fictionalized or composite illustrations created solely to demonstrate concepts and practices. They are not intended to represent, resemble, or refer to any actual person, living or deceased, or to any specific event, organization, or entity. Any similarity to real persons or events is coincidental and is not intended to harm, defame, or misrepresent any individual or group.

The author and publisher make no representations or warranties, express or implied, regarding the completeness, accuracy, reliability, or suitability of the information contained in this book. No specific outcomes are guaranteed. Results from the practices described will vary from person to person and depend on individual circumstances, consistency of practice, and many factors outside the scope of this book. Readers are fully responsible for their own decisions and actions, and any use of the information in this book is at the reader's own risk. Neither the author nor the publisher shall be held liable for any loss, injury, or damage, direct or indirect, arising from the use or misuse of the material herein.

First Edition

ISBN: 978-1-7646390-5-7

Table of Contents

Preface

Self-criticism is not just a thinking error. It is often a nervous-system strategy.

Most books on self-compassion treat the inner critic as a set of incorrect thoughts to be argued away with better counter-evidence. They rarely produce durable change. The reader with a loud critic has usually tried the counter-evidence, repeatedly, over years, and has found the critic present the following morning. The reason is not a lack of effort. The reason is that the critic is not, at its root, a thought at all. It is a physiological pattern shaped by an older emotional system, and that system does not respond to logic in the way a reasoning problem does.

The inner critic is a strategy of threat. It uses attack, shame, and contempt because, in the environment that shaped the human brain, these were among the fastest ways to force behavioral change and preserve belonging. Modern humans live in conditions the system was not built for, and the attacks now land on the person using them, producing depression, anxiety, physical exhaustion, and relational damage rather than safety. Understanding the critic in these terms changes the work. The critic becomes a system to be regulated, re-trained, and met with something older than itself. It is not a debate partner to be defeated.

Compassion Focused Therapy, developed in the United Kingdom by Paul Gilbert and extended over the past two decades by a broad clinical community, works directly with patterns of threat, safeness, and emotional regulation. It builds, in the reader, a second voice that speaks with wisdom, strength, warmth, and caring commitment. It does this through specific practices that can help strengthen the soothing system with consistent repetition. The evidence base for compassion-based interventions is now substantial, with reviews and meta-analyses reporting reductions in self-criticism, depression, anxiety, and shame, alongside gains in wellbeing and emotion regulation (Kirby et al., 2017).

Many readers arrive at this material after cognitive behavioral therapy has helped them partially but left the core self-criticism intact. Others come after years of positive-thinking strategies that produced temporary improvement and persistent relapse. Still others arrive without having tried formal therapy, drawn by a growing sense that the voice in their head is costing them more than they once recognized. All three groups will find the material addressed to them directly.

The pages ahead are written as a beginner's introduction, in plain American English, for readers without clinical training. Each chapter presents one piece of the model, supported by research, illustrated with real situations, and anchored in practices that can be started the day they are read. The practices are cumulative. The foundational ones introduced in Part Four are assumed in the chapters that follow, so the recommended path through the book is linear on a first reading and nonlinear on any reading after that.

By the end, the reader will have met the inner critic on different terms, will understand the three emotion systems that underlie most mental states, and will have a working relationship with five foundational CFT practices: soothing rhythm breathing, safe place imagery, the compassionate other, compassionate letter writing, and chair dialogue with the critic. The reader will also have a framework for integrating the work into daily life, for recognizing when older material surfaces during the practice, and for knowing when professional support should be sought. The closing chapters address the long arc of practice over years rather than weeks.

What follows is not a promise of rapid change. It is a foundation. Many readers notice meaningful shifts over time when they practice consistently, because the work is aimed at repeated emotional and physiological learning rather than momentary willpower. The chapters ahead are the path.

How To Use This Book

Read the book in order on a first pass. The chapters build on one another. The physiological framework in Part Two underlies everything that follows, and the foundational practices introduced in Part Four are referenced throughout Parts Five and Six. Skipping ahead to the practices without the framework tends to produce practice that does not stick, because the reader has no understanding of why the practice works or when to apply it.

After a first complete reading, the book becomes a reference. Return to individual chapters as specific questions arise. The chapter on the inner critic, the chapter on shame, and the chapter on backdraft are common re-read targets. The quick reference at the back of the book summarizes every practice in one place for fast lookup.

Plan for gradual progress. This work asks for repetition, and people differ in how quickly it starts to feel natural. Some readers notice early shifts within weeks; for others, it takes longer. What matters most is steady practice and realistic expectations.

If the material becomes difficult at any point, particularly in Chapter 16 on backdraft or Chapter 17 on working with a difficult past, slow the pace, reach for the simpler practices, and consider professional support. The closing sections of this book include specific guidance on when and how to seek help, along with directories of trained clinicians across the major English-speaking regions.

PART I: THE PROBLEM WE DO NOT TALK ABOUT

Chapter 1: The Voice That Tears You Down

Thomas closed his laptop at 3:42 p.m., and the room went still. The Zoom call was over. He had just given the quarterly update to about forty people, most of them senior to him. His heart was still beating fast. He had stumbled on one slide, had tripped over the name of a new client, and had finished the last point about thirty seconds late.

He sat for a moment. His coffee was cold. Outside, a lawnmower started somewhere down the street.

And then his mind started talking to him.

You are such an idiot. Forty people just watched you blank out on a client name you have seen a hundred times. Your boss is going to think you are not ready for this. You probably are not ready for this. Remember when Diego gave the presentation last quarter? He did not fumble once. He did not sweat through his shirt. What is wrong with you? You have been doing this for years and you still sound nervous. People can tell. They always can tell.

Twenty minutes later, Thomas was still sitting there. He had not moved. He had not sent the follow-up email he was supposed to send. He was still being lectured, and the lecturer was him.

By dinner, he had almost decided to ask for the next presentation to go to someone else. He would say he was too busy. He would say it was a development opportunity for someone junior. The real reason was sitting right there in his chest, but he did not want to name it, because naming it would make it worse.

What You'll Get From This Chapter

In the next few pages, you will meet the voice that has probably been running in the background of your mind for years. You will learn what it is, where it came from, and why it lies to you while sounding so convincing. You will see how it shows up in different forms, and how those forms all share a strange, misplaced sense of purpose. By the end, you will have one short exercise that takes about a day to complete and that can change, in a small but real way, how you experience your own thinking.

1.1 Meeting The Critic Head On

Most of us do not realize we have an inner critic until someone points it out. We think we are just thinking. The voice that tells us we are stupid, lazy, boring, ugly, or a failure feels like an observation, not a character in the room. It feels like *us* noticing a truth about ourselves.

It is not. It is a voice. It has patterns. It has favorite topics. It has a tone. It repeats itself. And once you learn to spot it, you will notice it everywhere.

The inner critic is the habitual pattern of self-attacking thought that shows up when you fail, when you feel exposed, when you compare yourself to others, or sometimes for no reason you can identify. Psychologists have been studying it for decades, and it has many names across different schools. Gilbert and Procter (2006) describe compassion-focused work as especially relevant for people whose difficulties are organized around shame and self-criticism. That detail matters. The critic is not evil. It is misguided.

You might think of it like a smoke alarm that went off once when you were eight, then never stopped. The alarm was real. The fire was real too. But the alarm has not learned that the fire is out.

1.2 Why It Feels Like Truth

One of the cruelest things about the inner critic is how much it sounds like reality. The voice does not say, "I am feeling anxious about that presentation, and I might be overestimating how badly it went." The voice says, "You are an idiot."

There is a reason this happens. Threat-based thoughts ride on strong emotion, and strong emotion makes thoughts feel more true. In cognitive therapy, this process is often described as emotional reasoning (Beck & Haigh, 2014). When you are anxious, anxious-flavored thoughts feel correct. When you are ashamed, shame-flavored thoughts feel correct. The felt sense of truth is not coming from the accuracy of the thought. It is coming from the intensity of the feeling underneath it.

Think of it this way. If you have ever been on a plane during turbulence and had the thought *this plane is going to crash*, you know that the thought felt absolutely real in the moment, even though the statistical chance of it being correct is very, very low. That is emotional reasoning. The fear makes the catastrophic thought feel like a prediction instead of a symptom.

The inner critic works the same way. It rides on shame, on fear, on the feeling of having been exposed. In that storm, the critic's statements feel like a neutral report. They are not. They are weather.

1.3 A Real Example

Gemma runs a small bakery in the front half of a coffee shop. She has been doing it for four years. The bakery is good. Customers tell her it is good. The shop next door refers people to her for wedding cakes.

One morning, she made a batch of croissants that came out too dark. Not burnt. Just darker than she wanted. She sold them anyway because the shop was busy, and three customers complimented them. One customer, the kind who wears expensive running gear and speaks in short sentences, said, "These are a little over done, aren't they?"

Gemma smiled, apologized, and offered a replacement. The customer declined and left.

By the end of the day, Gemma had replayed that moment forty times. In her head, the customer's comment was not a passing note about a single pastry. It was a judgment on her entire skill, her entire business, her entire decision to leave a stable office job to bake for a living. Her critic was loud. *You do not know what you are doing. You have been faking it this whole time. Everyone has been too polite to say so. This one was honest and now you know.*

What she tried was the usual move. She tried to argue with the critic. *The other customers liked them. The shop next door referred a bride to me last week. I have been doing this for four years.* Arguing, in the moment, did almost nothing. The critic kept going. That night, Gemma could not sleep.

What finally helped was not arguing. It was simply writing down what her critic had said, word for word, in her notebook. She was shocked when she read it back. She would never, ever, in a hundred years, say those things to another baker. She would not say them to a friend. She would not say them to a stranger. And yet they had been blasting through her head for hours.

What this means for you: Writing your critic down is one of the fastest ways to notice it is not a neutral report. It is a voice, and it speaks in a way you would not tolerate from anyone else.

1.4 The Forms It Takes

The critic shows up differently in different people. Gilbert and colleagues have identified several forms, and once you know them, you will recognize yours.

The Punitive Critic is loud and mean. It calls you names. It uses contempt. It is the voice that says things like *you are disgusting, you are stupid, you are pathetic.* People with punitive critics often grew up with someone who spoke to them this way, and they took the voice inside. The punitive critic is often linked to a form of shame Gilbert calls hated self, and it is the one most strongly associated with depression and self-harm (Gilbert et al., 2004).

The Perfectionist Critic is the one that never says good job. It moves the goalposts. When you finish something, it focuses on the part that could have been better. When you achieve something, it dismisses the achievement and points to the next one. It is often experienced as motivating, at first. Over time, it becomes the voice that runs people into burnout.

The Comparative Critic is always measuring. It scans for people who are thinner, richer, more successful, more loved, better parents, better writers, better anything. When it finds them, it uses them as evidence against you. Social media is rocket fuel for this one.

The Anxious Critic specializes in what-if. It reviews your decisions, your past conversations, your future plans, and it finds every place something could go wrong. It thinks it is helping you prepare. It is actually wearing you out.

Most people have a mix. One form tends to dominate, but others show up in specific situations. Noticing which form is running in a given moment is already a step toward separating from it.

1.5 Another Real Example

Kenji is fifty-one. He runs a small accounting practice. On paper, his life looks good. Wife, two adult kids, a house in a quiet suburb, a business that breaks even every year. He has never been diagnosed with depression or anxiety. He has never seen a therapist.

He also has not slept through the night in about a decade.

Around 3 a.m., almost every night, Kenji wakes up. What wakes him is a replay. A client he was short with. An email he wrote that came across wrong. A moment at the dinner table where his son looked irritated. A comment his wife made in the parking lot of a grocery store six years ago that he still thinks about.

His critic is not loud. It does not call him names. It is a patient, low, relentless reviewer. It gathers evidence that Kenji is letting people down, falling short, not doing enough, not being enough. Over the years, this voice has become so familiar that Kenji does not even hear it anymore. He just wakes up tired.

What he tried first was sleeping pills. They helped him stay asleep, but they did not stop the thoughts on the nights he did wake up. He tried meditation apps. He stopped after three weeks because, in his words, "I do not have a meditation kind of brain."

What finally started to shift things was a single question from his adult daughter, who was home for a weekend. She asked him, "Dad, do you know how hard you are on yourself?" He had not known. Not really. He had assumed that was just how thinking went. The question landed hard enough that he started, for the first time in his life, to pay attention to the voice in his head.

What this means for you: The critic does not always announce itself. Sometimes it has been with you so long you no longer recognize it as a voice. Sometimes you need someone who loves you to point at it before you can even see it.

1.6 The Misguided Protector

Here is the reframe that changes everything for most readers.

The inner critic is not your enemy. It is trying to protect you.

The punitive critic is trying to beat you to the punch. If it calls you stupid first, maybe nobody else will. If it tears your work apart before it is submitted, you can prepare for the worst. If you hate yourself before anyone else has a chance to, you will not be surprised by their rejection.

The perfectionist critic is trying to keep you safe through performance. If you are never good enough, you will never stop pushing. If you never stop pushing, you will never fall behind. If you never fall behind, you will not be exposed as the failure it secretly believes you are.

The comparative critic is trying to tell you what the group values so you will not be left out. It thinks that by pointing at the people who have more, it is keeping you motivated to earn your place.

The anxious critic is trying to catch the danger before it catches you.

Every form of the critic has a protective logic, even when the logic is wrong and the strategy is harmful. This matters because it changes the goal.

You are not trying to kill the critic. You are not trying to silence it. You are not trying to win a fight against it. You are trying to do two things. First, you are trying to see it clearly. Second, over time, you are trying to grow a different voice alongside it. A voice that has the protection job too, but does the job with warmth, strength, and wisdom instead of attack.

That other voice is what the rest of this book is about. But you cannot grow it until you can see what is currently standing in its place.

1.7 When It Doesn't Work

Some readers try the exercises in this chapter and feel worse, not better. That happens. Here is what is usually going on.

The most common trap is trying to fight the critic with logic. You write down what the critic said. Then you immediately write a rebuttal underneath it. Then the critic comes back with a counter-argument. Then you counter-counter. Two hours later you are exhausted, the critic has won, and you are now also mad at yourself for not being able to win an argument with your own mind.

This is not the exercise working wrong. It is the exercise being misused. The point is not to argue with the critic. The point is to notice it and name it.

Three things to try if this happens:

1. Stop writing the rebuttal. Just write the critic's lines and nothing else. The act of transcription creates space. You do not need to add anything.

2. Read what you wrote out loud. Hearing the critic in your own voice, spoken into a quiet room, changes how seriously you take it. Many readers start laughing, or crying, or both. The spell breaks for a moment.

3. Show one sentence to a trusted person. Just one. Ask them, "Is this true?" Hearing someone you love say "no" is often worth a hundred internal rebuttals.

If none of that helps, and if your critic seems to be attached to memories of actual abuse, please move carefully. Set this book down and consider reaching out to a therapist. There is no prize for powering through. The critic will still be here in two weeks.

1.8 The Quick Version

You have an inner critic. Almost everyone does. It is a pattern of self-attacking thought that feels like truth but is not. It sounds neutral, but if you write it down, you will see how cruel it actually is.

The critic takes different forms: punitive, perfectionist, comparative, anxious. Most people have a primary form with secondary ones that show up in specific situations. Identifying your primary form is useful for later chapters.

The most important idea in this chapter is the reframe: the critic is a misguided protector, not an enemy. It grew out of some combination of inherited voices, past hurts, and a survival instinct that never got updated. Fighting it directly does not work. Seeing it clearly does.

Your job this week is simple. For one day, carry a small notebook or use the notes app on your phone. Every time you catch your critic speaking, write the exact words down. Do not argue with them. Do not add commentary. Just record. Before you go to bed that night, read the list back to yourself.

Most readers are shocked by what they find. Some are moved to tears. Some laugh. Some feel a quiet anger, not at themselves, but at the voice that has been running in the background for years.

Any of those responses is fine. The point is to see. Once you can see, you can start to work with it, and that work begins in the chapters ahead.

Chapter 2: Shame Wants You to Hide

Fatima stood on the sidewalk outside her friend's apartment, her hand hovering near the buzzer. She had known about the party for three weeks. She had bought a bottle of wine, chosen an outfit, cancelled twice in her head, and then talked herself into going. She could hear laughter and music through the second-floor window. Someone was telling a story and everyone was cracking up.

She did not press the buzzer.

She stood there for maybe four minutes, telling herself she needed to just do it, and feeling her body do the opposite. Her chest got tight. Her face got warm. Her feet felt heavy. It was not quite fear, not in the way she felt fear at a job interview or before a flight. It was something older and more physical. Something that wanted her to leave. Something that wanted her to disappear.

She texted her friend that her stomach had suddenly turned, that she was so sorry, that she would call tomorrow. Then she walked back to her car, holding the unopened bottle of wine, and drove home.

On the drive, she did not cry. She did not feel sad, exactly. She felt something hotter and heavier than sadness. She kept seeing herself through imagined eyes, standing in the doorway of a room full of people, being clocked as awkward, unfunny, badly dressed, forgettable. She had been doing this for decades. Canceling, withdrawing, hiding. She did not know it had a name.

What You'll Get From This Chapter

This chapter is about the single most painful emotion most readers of this book live with, and most readers do not know it by its proper name. You will learn what shame actually is, how it differs from guilt in ways that change everything, why it is the emotion that drives so much of what your critic does, and where you can expect to feel it in your body. By the end, you will be able to recognize shame in real time, which is the first step toward not being run by it.

2.1 Shame Is Not Guilt

If you take only one thing from this chapter, take this one. **Shame and guilt are not the same emotion.** They feel similar. They get lumped together in everyday language. Therapists sometimes use them interchangeably. They are different, and the difference matters.

Guilt is the feeling you get when you think *I did a bad thing.* It points at a specific action. It is uncomfortable, but it is workable. If you feel guilty for snapping at your partner, guilt pushes you toward an apology, a repair, a different behavior next time. Guilt, in research and in lived experience, is actually associated with healthier outcomes. It motivates change without attacking who you are (Tangney et al., 2007).

Shame is the feeling you get when you think *I am a bad thing.* It does not point at a specific action. It points at your whole self. It says, *there is something wrong with me at the core, as a person, and if people really knew, they would recoil.* Shame is existential. Guilt is behavioral.

Picture the difference this way. Two people spill coffee on a stranger's shirt.

Person one thinks, "That was careless. I should apologize and offer to pay for the cleaning." They feel embarrassed. They feel bad. They feel motivated to repair. That is guilt.

Person two thinks, "Oh my God, I am such a disaster. Why can I not do anything right. This is exactly the kind of thing that happens to me. Everyone is looking." They feel hot, small, and desperate to leave. They want to vanish. That is shame.

Both people spilled the same coffee. The first person is going to buy some club soda and move on. The second person is going to replay the incident at 2 a.m. for three nights. Same event, two very different emotional responses, two very different outcomes.

This is why shame is so much more damaging than guilt. Guilt looks at the action and asks for a correction. Shame looks at the self and asks for erasure.

2.2 Two Kinds Of Shame

Gilbert makes a further distinction that most readers find useful. He splits shame into two kinds (Gilbert, 2003).

External shame is about how you believe you appear in the minds of others. It is the sense that other people see you as inadequate, unlikeable, inferior, or disgusting. You do not need evidence. You can be at a coffee shop, look up, and simply feel that the stranger in line behind you is judging you. External shame is the driver behind most social anxiety, much of the discomfort of walking into a new group, and the specific dread of being watched.

Internal shame is how you see yourself. It is the felt belief that you are not okay at the level of your own self-evaluation. It is the mirror moment when you look at your own reflection and feel something close to disgust. It is the way you can be alone in your house, with no one watching, and still feel shame.

Most people with a serious shame problem have both kinds, and the two feed each other. You believe others see you as defective, so you start to see yourself that way. Or you believe you are defective, and you assume everyone else must be seeing it too. Gilbert's research suggests that internal shame is actually the more stubborn of the two, because it does not need external input. It runs on its own fuel (Matos & Pinto-Gouveia, 2010).

Fatima, standing outside her friend's apartment, was running on both. She was certain she would appear awkward and forgettable in the room (external). She also believed, in some deep place she would not say out loud, that she actually was those things (internal). That combination produced the hot, heavy immobility that kept her from pressing the buzzer.

2.3 A Real Example

Diego was at a dinner party. He said something in response to a comment about local politics. He did not think much of it while saying it. He was trying to be funny. It was not funny. A small silence followed. Someone changed the subject.

That was it. The whole event took about eight seconds.

By the time Diego was driving home, he had replayed the moment about thirty times. Each replay got worse. His brain added things. *They all thought I was stupid. They all thought I was trying too hard. They are going to talk about it after I leave. They are talking about it now. I should not have gone. I am always like this at these things.*

By the time he got home, he was sitting in his car in the driveway with the engine off, unable to go inside. His body felt heavy. His face was hot. He had been crying at some point on the drive and could not remember when he had started.

What he tried first was distraction. He went inside, put on a show, scrolled his phone. The replays kept coming. He tried texting his best friend to complain about the party, hoping for sympathy. His friend responded supportively, but the moment his friend's message arrived, Diego felt even worse. He could hear his critic saying, *now you are bothering him too.*

What finally helped, though it took two more days, was one small realization. His wife, who had been at the same dinner, told him over breakfast, "That comment you made? I do not even remember it. I remember the pasta." He almost cried again. Not because he had been wrong to feel bad, but because he realized how much of his suffering had been about an event that, for everyone else, had evaporated.

What this means for you: Shame has a strong tendency to act as if the event is still happening in everyone else's mind, long after it has left the room. The first step is noticing that the story your shame is telling is probably not the story anyone else is living.

2.4 Shame In The Body

Shame is not just a thought. It is a physical event. If you pay attention, you can often feel it before you can name it.

Common physical signs of shame include: A hot or flushing sensation in the face, ears, or neck, A heavy weight in the chest or stomach, The feeling of being small, as if you want to shrink, A sudden drop in energy, almost like being pushed down, An urge to hide your face, look at the floor, or cover your body, and A frozen quality, as if you cannot move or speak.

There is a reason for all of this. Shame is an old emotion. It evolved in social animals (including humans) as a signal that your standing in the group might be at risk (Gilbert, 2003). The physical signs of shame, the slumping, the looking down, the hiding, are what psychologists call submissive displays. They are the body's way of saying *I am not a threat, please do not push me out*. They worked for our ancestors, because staying in the group meant surviving.

They do not work as well for you, sitting on a couch replaying a comment from a dinner party. But the body does not know that. The body runs the old program.

This is why trying to think your way out of shame rarely works. Shame lives below language. You have to reach it through the body before thoughts can get a foothold. That is part of why the practices in Part Four of this book focus so heavily on breath, posture, and imagery. They are aimed at the place shame actually lives.

2.5 Another Real Example

Elena, thirty-seven, avoided mirrors. Not in an obvious way. She had mirrors in her bathroom and her bedroom. She used them. But she used them fast, in and out, without lingering. She did not take selfies. She rarely looked at photos of herself. When friends posted group shots, she scrolled past quickly.

One evening, she was getting ready for a friend's birthday dinner. She put on an outfit she liked, did her makeup, and then, on impulse, stopped and actually looked. Really looked. Not the glance. The full look.

And something caught her off guard. She started to cry. Not sad crying. Something more specific. A grief, almost. She could not fully see herself in the mirror. She could see her face, her body, her clothes, but she could also feel a familiar overlay, a kind of running commentary in her head that had been going on so long she did not even notice it anymore. The commentary was cataloging. The skin. The line of the nose. The way one eye sits a little lower than the other. The belly. The arms. Every detail, noted and filed as evidence.

She had lived inside that overlay her entire adult life. She had never seen her own face without it.

What she tried, without fully knowing why, was simply to stand there. She did not argue with the commentary. She did not try to silence it. She just let it run, and she stayed with the reflection, and she breathed. After a few minutes, something loosened. Not completely. Not for good. But for a moment, she saw a face, not a list of flaws. It was the face of a person who had been tired for a long time. The person in the mirror looked like someone who needed kindness, not another review.

She went to the dinner. She did not tell anyone about the moment in front of the mirror. But something small had shifted.

What this means for you: Internal shame often lives in specific places in your life. A mirror. A swimsuit. A voice memo of yourself. The place where it lives is a clue. And sometimes, simply staying with the place (without fighting it, without fleeing it) is the first crack in the wall.

2.6 Why Shame Feels So Heavy

Shame's weight is not in your imagination. Research has linked chronic shame to depression, anxiety disorders, eating disorders, addiction, trauma-related symptoms, and suicidality (Kim et al., 2011). It is one of the most psychologically corrosive emotions we have, and yet it is rarely talked about by name, which is part of why it stays so powerful.

Shame thrives in silence. The less we name it, the more it grows. Most readers of this book have gone their whole lives feeling something heavy, painful, and isolating without ever learning the word for it. Getting the word is not a small thing. Research suggests that simply naming an emotion helps regulate it (Lieberman et al., 2007). Calling shame *shame* takes away some of its power.

The other reason shame feels so heavy is its social nature. Shame is not just about you. It is about you in the presence of others, real or imagined. Even when you are alone, the shame voice is speaking as if someone is watching. That imagined audience is what makes shame so exhausting. You are constantly performing for a room that is not there.

One way to think about it: guilt is uncomfortable but clean. You feel bad, you act to repair, you move on. Shame is uncomfortable and tangled. It tells you that the problem is who you are, which is not something you can repair through action, which is why shame leads so often to avoidance, hiding, numbing, or attacking yourself.

The good news is this: shame is treatable. It responds, slowly but reliably, to the kind of work CFT was built to do. You are not stuck with it forever. You are not too far gone. Research on compassion-based and CFT-informed interventions reports reductions in shame and self-criticism across a range of populations (Gilbert & Procter, 2006; Kirby et al., 2017).

Nothing in this paragraph is meant to minimize how hard it is. Only to give you information: the thing you have been carrying has a name, it has a mechanism, and it has a treatment. That alone is worth something.

2.7 When It Doesn't Work

Some readers try to name shame in their lives and cannot find it. They feel bad, they know they feel bad, but they cannot seem to locate the specific emotion. Others feel so much shame when they try to name it that they have to put the book down.

Both experiences are normal. Here is what to do.

If you cannot find shame in yourself, that is information, not failure. Shame is often buried under other emotions. You might feel anger first (at yourself or at others). You might feel numbness. You might feel tiredness. Those can all be shame wearing a different coat. Spend a few days simply noticing when you feel the urge to hide, to avoid, to cancel plans, to go silent, or to leave. That urge is often where shame lives, even when the emotion itself is not consciously present.

If naming shame makes you feel worse, that is also information, and it is worth taking seriously. Three things to try:

1. Slow down. Read this chapter in smaller chunks. Spread it over a week. There is no prize for finishing it fast.

2. Pair the reading with something soothing. A cup of tea. A warm room. A pet nearby. The body needs grounding when the content is heavy.

3. Talk to one trusted person about what you are reading. Not to be fixed. Just to be heard. Shame loses weight when it is spoken out loud to someone safe.

If the feelings coming up feel unmanageable (if old memories are flooding in, if you feel panicked or dissociated, if you are thinking about harming yourself), please stop and reach out to a mental health professional. A book is not the right tool for you at this moment. A human being is.

2.8 What To Take Away

Shame is the emotion that wants you hidden. It tells you that the problem is not something you did but something you are. It is different from guilt, it is heavier, and it is the driver behind much of what your inner critic does.

Shame comes in two flavors: external (how you believe you appear to others) and internal (how you see yourself). Most people with a serious shame problem carry both, and they reinforce each other.

Shame is a physical event as much as a thought. It shows up in the body as heat, heaviness, shrinking, and the urge to hide. That physical quality is why thinking alone does not touch it. The body has to be part of the work, which is why the practices in later chapters will involve breath, posture, and imagery.

Shame is common, shame is treatable, and shame loses some of its power the moment you give it its right name. For the rest of this week, your job is to notice. Not fix. Not argue. Just notice. When do you feel the urge to hide? When do you go quiet? When do you cancel? When do you look away from your own reflection? Each noticing is a small act of turning on the lights in a room that has been dark for a long time.

In the next chapter, we look at what all this costs, not to pile on pain, but to clarify why a different approach is worth trying.

Chapter 3: The Real Cost Of Self Attack

Raj is forty-four. He has been hard on himself for as long as he can remember. Genuinely hard. The voice in his head has been running since he was about nine, when his father, a kind but distant man, once said, "We work twice as hard because we have to." Raj took that on like a uniform and never took it off.

By the time he sat down across from his doctor this past January, he had three things going on. His blood pressure was high enough that the doctor wanted to start medication. His sleep was broken; he slept about five hours a night and had for years. And his wife had told him the previous weekend, in a careful, quiet tone, that she felt lonely in their marriage.

On paper, Raj's life looked great. Good job. Two good kids. A house he owned. A wife who still wanted to work things out, even after the lonely conversation. He did not drink too much. He did not smoke. He had never had an affair. He had never been fired.

Inside, he was running on fumes, and he did not know why.

What his doctor said was the first thing that stopped him. "Your labs are not that bad. But your face is. You look like a man who has not been nice to himself in a long time."

Raj laughed. Then, unexpectedly, in a sterile exam room under fluorescent light, he cried.

What You'll Get From This Chapter

This chapter is about the accumulating price of chronic self-attack. Not in a scare-tactic way. In an honest, research-backed way. You will see what self-criticism and shame do over years to your mood, your sleep and body, your ambitions, and your relationships. You will see why the critic, for all its claims of protecting you, actually undermines almost everything it says it is trying to save. And you will get a first glimpse of why a different approach is not only possible but, according to decades of research, more effective than the one you have been running.

3.1 The Cost To Your Mood

Self-criticism is a well-established correlate and risk factor in depression research. Reviews suggest that people who score higher in self-critical thinking are more likely to report depressive symptoms and broader psychopathology, and they may respond less well to treatment than people with lower scores (Blatt, 2004; Werner et al., 2019).

Let that sentence do its work for a moment. This is not a vague association. The research is clear and repeated. When the self-critic runs loud, mood suffers. Not as a mystery. As a mechanism.

Here is how the mechanism may work. The critic feeds you a stream of threat-based information: you are failing, you are not enough, you should have done better, people are disappointed in you. Your body does not fully distinguish between an external threat and an internally generated social-evaluative threat. To your nervous system, a mind flooded with critical thoughts can look a lot like an environment that is unsafe. Stress physiology stays activated. Over time, mood can sink, motivation can drop, and the capacity to feel pleasure can narrow.

It gets worse. When the critic triggers low mood, the low mood itself becomes new ammunition for the critic. *Now you are sad too. What is wrong with you? Snap out of it.* This is what Shahar (2015) called the self-critical cascade: the critic creates distress, the distress becomes evidence for the critic, and the loop spins faster. Many people who end up in depression describe this exact pattern without knowing its name.

Anxiety follows a similar path. The constant sense of being judged by your own mind keeps the threat system engaged. Your baseline stress rises. Sleep suffers. Decision-making gets harder. The small worries that most people shake off start to feel unbearable. High self-criticism is a strong predictor of generalized anxiety, social anxiety, and panic (Werner et al., 2019).

The cruel part is that the critic thinks it is helping. It thinks it is keeping you sharp, keeping you ahead, keeping you safe. It is actually burning out the exact systems you need to be sharp, ahead, and safe.

3.2 The Cost To Your Body

Your mind and your body are not two things. This is obvious when you say it, and strangely easy to forget when you live it. Chronic self-criticism does not stay in the brain. It shows up in the body, in ways you can measure.

Research on self-criticism has linked it to:

Poor sleep quality and insomnia. People with loud inner critics often cannot fall asleep, cannot stay asleep, or wake early with replaying thoughts (Ehret et al., 2015).

Stress linked to shame and social-evaluative threat has also been associated with inflammatory responses in laboratory and clinical research, which may help explain part of the wear-and-tear people feel when they live under chronic self-attack (Dickerson et al., 2009).

Digestive issues. The gut is one of the first places chronic stress shows up. Bloating, reflux, irritable bowel symptoms, and appetite changes all track with high baseline threat activation.

Tension patterns. Jaw clenching, shoulder tightness, low back pain, and tension headaches often have a self-criticism component that nobody is looking for.

Raj's high blood pressure did not appear out of nowhere. It appeared after thirty-five years of a pressurized inner life. His doctor, to his credit, was looking at more than the numbers on the chart.

The body keeps the score, as one well-known book title puts it. The inner critic is not free. It is costing you, every day, in ways you might be writing off as stress, aging, or bad genes. Those are often part of the picture. But a loud, chronic critic is often the part of the picture that nobody is talking about.

3.3 A Real Example

Maria is fifty-two. She runs a mid-sized marketing firm. For the last eight years, she has slept about four to five hours a night. She has tried magnesium, melatonin, weighted blankets, lavender, sleep tracking apps, cutting caffeine, yoga, a memory foam mattress, and a prescription sleep aid her doctor eventually refused to renew. Nothing has really worked for more than a week or two.

The pattern is always the same. She falls asleep fine. She wakes around 2:30 or 3:00 a.m. She reaches for her phone. She starts reviewing. Yesterday's meetings. Tomorrow's meetings. A comment she made three weeks ago. A staff member she should have managed differently. By 4:30 a.m. she is exhausted but wide awake, furious at herself for not being able to sleep, which makes her less able to sleep.

What she tried first was better sleep hygiene. The dark room. The phone out of the bedroom. The bedtime routine. Some of this helped on the margins. The 3 a.m. reviewing did not stop. It just happened in the dark, staring at the ceiling, instead of on her phone.

What shifted things was not a sleep intervention at all. It was six weeks of working with a therapist on self-criticism. She did not focus on sleep during those sessions. She focused on the voice that had been running the 3 a.m. review for eight years. When the voice quieted down, even partially, the sleep followed. Not fully. Not every night. But enough that her doctor stopped suggesting a formal sleep study.

What this means for you: If you have a physical symptom that has not responded to physical treatments, the problem may not be physical. Or, more accurately, the physical problem may have a psychological engine underneath it. Chronic self-criticism is one of the most common engines, and treating it often relieves symptoms that a hundred supplements could not touch.

3.4 The Cost To Your Relationships

This is often the cost that surprises people the most. You would think that the people who are hard on themselves would be gentle with others, since they know how much being judged hurts. Sometimes that is true. Often, it is not.

Chronic self-criticism tends to leak outward. It shows up as:

Difficulty receiving care. When someone tries to comfort you, thank you, or compliment you, you deflect. You do not trust it. You change the subject. The person trying to care for you learns, over time, that their care does not land, and they stop offering it.

Hyper-vigilance to judgment. You assume others are judging you the way you judge yourself. You read subtle cues where none exist. You misread neutral expressions as disapproval. Your friends and partner feel they have to walk on eggshells.

Defensive responses to feedback. Because any criticism lands on top of an already-critical inner voice, even gentle feedback feels like an attack. You defend, withdraw, or lash out. The people around you learn to stop giving you honest information.

Projected harshness. Some self-critics become critical of others. If your standards for yourself are impossible, your standards for the people around you often become impossible too. This is one of the least talked about consequences of a loud inner critic, and one of the most damaging to long-term relationships.

Emotional unavailability. When you are constantly managing your own inner storm, there is not much bandwidth left for being present with the people you love. You are there, but you are not there.

Raj's wife did not say he was a bad husband. She said she felt lonely. Those two things are different, and the difference is important. She was not accusing. She was describing. A man who spends most of his inner life in a silent argument with himself has limited capacity to be with anyone else, even the person sleeping next to him.

3.5 Another Real Example

James teaches high school English. He is beloved by his students. He has been teaching for fifteen years, has won a district award, and has been recommended for department chair twice. He turned it down both times.

His critic is the perfectionist kind. Every lesson could have been better. Every essay he graded, he graded wrong in some way.

Every parent conversation, he replayed in his head with the things he should have said. When he is praised, he feels embarrassed, because he knows how much he is falling short. When he is criticized, even mildly, he spirals for days.

His marriage of twelve years ended three years ago. When his ex-partner finally explained it, in the quiet way people explain things that have been building for years, she said: "I feel like I have been dating your disapproval of yourself."

James did not understand that sentence at first. He thought she meant he had been depressed, which he had not been, not really. It took him a year and two different therapists to hear what she had actually said. He had been so consumed with managing his own internal disappointment that his partner had been left to love him alone. She had been in the relationship with his critic, not with him. Eventually, that relationship ended, because no one can be in love with a person who is mostly not there.

What he tried next is what this book is about. He did not try to fix his relationships first. He started, slowly, with the voice. He began noticing it. Naming it. Writing it down. Only months later, almost as a side effect, did he realize that he was actually listening when his new partner spoke. He was there. He could receive her comment about the soup being good without immediately cataloging all the ways it could have been better. Something had rearranged.

What this means for you: If your relationships are strained in ways you cannot quite name, the problem may not be them. It may not even be you, exactly. It may be your critic, occupying space that should belong to the people you love.

3.6 A Different Approach Is Possible

Here is the reframe that changes everything for most readers of this book.

You do not have to choose between self-criticism and falling apart. That is the false choice the critic sells. It tells you that if you let it go, you will become lazy, arrogant, sloppy, mediocre, or out of control. It tells you it is the only thing standing between you and the worst version of yourself.

The research points in the opposite direction. People who develop self-compassion do not simply drop their standards. Across the literature, self-compassion is associated with healthier motivation, greater persistence after setbacks, and a more constructive response to personal failure (Neff, 2003; Terry & Leary, 2011). They do not become lazy. They become more able to take on hard things, because they are no longer paralyzed by the fear of failure. They do not become arrogant. They become more honest about their flaws, because they are less defended against them.

The critic is not the engine of your competence. Your competence is the engine of your competence. Your kindness, your skill, your curiosity, your care, your experience, these are what actually produce good work. The critic has been taking credit for what the rest of you has been doing, and charging a tax that you have been paying in your mood, your sleep, your body, and your relationships.

You can let the tax go. That is what the rest of this book is about.

A different approach is not only possible. It exists, it has been studied for over two decades, and it has helped thousands of people who were exactly where you are right now. It is not a trick.

It is not a reframe. It is a slow, patient, physical, emotional, learnable set of skills.

Gilbert called the approach Compassion Focused Therapy because the word compassion was the best word available for what it is trying to grow inside you. A voice that is strong, wise, warm, and committed to your wellbeing. A voice that takes your suffering seriously. A voice that does not collapse under pressure. A voice that holds you to your values without holding you in contempt.

That voice can be grown. It is not a gift some people were born with and others were not. It is a skill, like riding a bike. Awkward at first. Strange-feeling. Then, slowly, natural.

Part Two of this book is where the building begins.

3.7 When It Doesn't Work

Some readers finish this chapter and feel more hopeful. Some finish it and feel worse, because the list of costs lands as one more thing to feel bad about. *Great. Now I am self-critical and my sleep is ruined and my marriage is strained. Add it to the pile.*

If that is what happened for you, please read what follows carefully.

This chapter is not a list of things you have done wrong. It is a list of things the critic has done to you. You did not choose to develop a loud inner critic. You did not choose to have it harm your sleep. You did not choose to have it leak into your relationships. It happened to you, often starting in childhood, often in ways you had no control over. The costs described in this chapter are not charges against your character. They are a description of what a long-running critic does, to anyone it inhabits.

Three things to try if this chapter has landed hard:

1. Take a day off. Do not open the book for twenty-four hours. Let the content settle. Some ideas need sleep before they finish their work.

2. Write down one cost that surprised you. Just one. Not a plan to fix it. Just the recognition. Recognition, without a demand to do something about it, is a gentler entry point than action.

3. Talk to one person you trust about what you are reading. Not to get advice. Just to say it out loud. Costs get lighter when they are shared with safe company.

If the chapter has triggered a significant emotional response (if you feel hopeless, if you are thinking about harming yourself, if you feel unable to function), please reach out to a mental health professional today. A book cannot carry you through a crisis. A human being can.

3.8 Wrapping Up

Chronic self-criticism and shame carry costs that accumulate over years. They show up in your mood, increasing the likelihood and severity of depression and anxiety. They show up in your body, as poor sleep, high baseline stress, and sometimes in physical symptoms that seem to resist other treatments. They show up in your ambitions, keeping you from taking on the things you are actually capable of. They show up in your relationships, leaking outward as defensiveness, emotional absence, and a strange difficulty in receiving care.

The critic claims it is protecting you. It is actually eroding you. The research on this is clear, and the pattern is consistent across populations and decades.

The good news is real. None of this is permanent. Self-criticism and shame respond to treatment. People who learn compassion-based skills see measurable reductions in depression, anxiety, shame, and self-attack, along with improvements in sleep, relationships, and overall life satisfaction (Kirby et al., 2017). This is not a miracle. It is a slow, steady shift, built from small daily practices done over weeks and months.

You have just finished the hardest part of the book. Part One names the problem. The rest of the book is about the answer.

In Part Two, you will meet the three-systems model. It is the single most useful piece of conceptual work in all of CFT. It will give you a way to understand your own mind that does not involve blame, and once you have it, nothing about your inner life will look quite the same again.

Take a breath. Take a break if you need one. When you are ready, turn the page.

PART II: HOW THE MIND AND BODY ACTUALLY WORK

Chapter 4: Your Brain Is Not Broken

Amara sat in the parking lot outside the urgent care, watching rain hit her windshield. Twenty minutes ago, she had been at a work lunch. She had taken one bite of a chicken wrap, felt a weird tingling in her left hand, and her mind had immediately gone to stroke. Heart attack. Blood clot. Something bad. Her chest started pounding. She could not breathe well. She excused herself, drove to the urgent care, checked in, got her vitals taken, and was told she was fine. The tingling was probably a pinched nerve from the way she had been sitting.

Fine. Physically fine. But on the drive back, she was not fine. She was furious. Not at the clinic. At herself.

What is wrong with you. You are a thirty-four year old woman having a panic attack over a tingling hand. You are falling apart. Other people do not do this. You are broken in some basic way and you have been broken for years and now it is getting worse.

She sat in the parking lot for a long time. Rain on the windshield. Her hands gripping the steering wheel. Her mind telling her that the problem was her, at the level of who she was as a person.

Nothing in that moment told her the actual truth. Which is that her brain had done exactly what brains evolved to do. A small sensation in her body had triggered an ancient threat detection system that was built to keep her ancestors alive when predators were real and clinics did not exist. The system had no way to tell a pinched nerve from a heart attack. It sounded the alarm. She felt afraid. Her body mobilized. And because she lives in a world where no actual lion was chasing her, the whole experience felt senseless, shameful, and like evidence that something was wrong with her.

Nothing was wrong with her. Her brain was doing its job. Her brain's job is just kind of poorly suited to modern life.

What You'll Get From This Chapter

This chapter introduces one of the most freeing ideas in CFT: your brain is not broken, it is just old. You will learn why humans inherited a mind that is prone to anxiety, self-criticism, and shame. You will see how that inheritance is the reason so much of what you struggle with is common, not personal. By the end, you will understand the difference between something being your fault and something being your responsibility, and why that distinction changes everything about how you approach the work ahead.

4.1 An Old Brain In A New World

Your brain is the product of about two million years of human evolution. Before that, it was built on the brains of earlier primates, and before that, on the brains of mammals that lived alongside dinosaurs. Every layer of your brain was shaped by a specific set of problems that our ancestors needed to survive.

Those problems were not the problems you have today. Your ancestors needed to spot predators in tall grass. They needed to find food when food was scarce. They needed to stay close to their tribe, because being cast out of the group was a death sentence. They needed to watch for signs of disease in other humans, because disease was one of the leading causes of death. They needed to remember threats with painful precision, because forgetting a threat could kill you.

All of those survival tools are still running in your head right now. They are the reason your heart pounds when a stranger looks at you too long in a grocery store. They are the reason one critical comment at work stays with you for six weeks while ten compliments evaporate by Tuesday. They are the reason social rejection feels like a physical wound. They are the reason you cannot sleep after an awkward conversation.

Paul Gilbert calls this the "tricky brain" problem (Gilbert, 2009). You have inherited a brain that was built for a world that no longer exists. You have also inherited newer capacities, including language, self-reflection, and the ability to imagine the future. Those newer capacities turn out to be incredibly useful for building civilization and writing books. They also turn out to be incredibly useful for generating anxiety, shame, and self-criticism, because you can now mentally simulate every possible way something could go wrong.

Put simply, the old brain cannot tell the difference between a real threat and an imagined one. Your newer brain can imagine endless threats. The result is a system that is always a little bit on fire, even when your actual life is safe.

4.2 Three Layers Stacked On Top Of Each Other

One useful way to think about the brain is as three rough layers, each built on top of the previous one. Neuroscientists do not treat this as a precise map of the brain, and the actual anatomy is far more interconnected than the clean picture suggests. Still, the rough layout can be a useful teaching tool when it is used as a metaphor rather than a literal model (MacLean, 1990; Haidt, 2006).

The oldest layer is sometimes called the reptilian brain. It handles survival basics: breathing, heart rate, flight or fight responses. It is fast, automatic, and not available for discussion. When you jerk your hand away from a hot pan before you have consciously registered the heat, that is this layer at work.

The middle layer, sometimes called the mammalian or emotional brain, developed to handle social behavior, attachment, and emotion. It gives you the ability to bond with your children, feel grief when someone dies, get angry when someone takes your lunch, and feel comforted when someone hugs you. This layer is where the three circles model of emotion, which you will meet in the next chapter, lives.

The newest layer is the cortex, especially the prefrontal cortex. This is the planning, reflecting, reasoning part of the brain. It is what lets you think about tomorrow, weigh options, write essays, and have opinions about opinions. It is also what lets you ruminate about a conversation you had in 2011.

The problem is that these three layers do not always cooperate. Your newest brain might know that the tingling in your hand is probably a pinched nerve. Your middle brain, fueled by your oldest brain, decides it is a heart attack. The newer brain gets outvoted. You end up in a parking lot in the rain.

This is not a defect. This is the mind you were given.

4.3 A Real Example

Ravi is thirty-nine, a software developer. He has a good job, a stable income, and a supportive partner. He has also, for as long as he can remember, felt vaguely uneasy almost all the time. Not anxious enough to be disabling. Just a low hum of not-quite-safe.

For years, he assumed this was a personality flaw. He tried meditation apps. He tried journaling. He tried therapy briefly, decided he was not making progress fast enough, and quit. He read books on anxiety and felt worse, because he did not match the profiles in the books. He did not have panic attacks. He did not have a specific phobia. He just felt off.

The thing that helped him was not a technique. It was a single paragraph he read in a book about evolution, which said something close to: humans evolved to always keep a little watch running in the background, because ancestors who stayed alert lived longer than ancestors who relaxed. Relaxation was a luxury. Alertness was survival. Modern humans are descended from the nervous ones.

Ravi read that paragraph three times. Then he closed the book and sat on his couch for about an hour, crying in a way he did not fully understand. For forty years, he had believed that his baseline unease was evidence that something was wrong with him. In one afternoon, he saw it for what it was. A feature, not a bug. An inheritance, not a flaw. His baseline tension was the price of being descended from survivors.

Nothing in his daily life changed overnight. But something more important changed. He stopped being angry at himself for feeling the way he felt. He had not been broken. He had been human.

What this means for you: Some of what you have been treating as a personal failing is simply the human condition. The low hum of unease, the tendency to watch for danger, the difficulty relaxing, the replay of old mistakes, these are things your ancestors passed down to you because they worked. They are not signs of failure. They are signs of lineage.

4.4 Not Your Fault, But Your Responsibility

Here is one of the most important ideas in CFT, and one of the ideas readers most often miss on the first read. Please slow down on this one.

The way your brain works is not your fault. You did not design it. You did not choose the emotional systems you inherited. You did not pick your temperament. You did not select your early attachment experiences. You did not decide which neural pathways would get reinforced in your first five years of life. Much of what drives your inner life was handed to you by biology and circumstance.

And.

It is still your responsibility. Not in a guilty way. In a practical way. Nobody else can do the work of learning to live with the brain you have. Your parents cannot do it. Your partner cannot do it. A therapist can help, but a therapist cannot actually reach into your mind and change your patterns for you. The work, slow and patient, is yours.

This is where a lot of self-help writing gets it wrong. Some books lean too hard on the fault side, implying that if you are suffering, you must be doing something wrong, and if you would just try harder or think differently, you could fix it. That framing produces more shame and less change. Other books lean too hard on the not-your-fault side, implying that because your suffering is not your fault, there is nothing you need to do about it except perhaps blame your childhood or your genes or the culture. That framing produces understanding without movement.

CFT holds both ideas at once. Your brain is not your fault. Your brain is your responsibility. Both sentences are true. Both sentences matter. If you collapse one into the other, you lose the whole point.

For Amara in the parking lot, this distinction is the gap between two futures. In one future, she keeps beating herself up for having a mind that panics over small sensations, and the panic gets worse, because shame feeds threat. In the other future, she learns to say to herself, "This is my brain doing what brains do. Now, here is what I can do about it." That second sentence is where all the work lives.

4.5 Another Real Example

Carlos is fifty-six. For most of his adult life, he has battled what he calls his "bad moods." Long stretches of low energy, self-criticism, and the feeling that nothing he did mattered. He had seen two therapists over the years. Both had suggested medication. Both had nudged him toward examining his childhood. Neither had worked. Carlos stopped going.

The thing that changed his relationship with his own mind was, of all things, a conversation with his grandson. Carlos was teaching the boy how to cast a fishing line. The boy got frustrated after the first few tries and threw the rod down, saying, "I am bad at this. I am just bad at stuff."

Carlos heard his own inner voice in his grandson's words. It stopped him cold. He sat the boy down on the dock and said something he did not plan. He said, "No, you are not bad at stuff. You are a new person learning a hard thing. Your hands do not know how to do this yet. That is not a flaw. That is a fact. We are going to teach your hands."

Later that night, Carlos could not stop thinking about what he had said. The kindness he had offered his grandson was kindness he had never, once, offered himself. He had treated every difficulty in his life as evidence of his own badness. His grandson, eight years old, had gotten more compassion from him in five seconds than Carlos had gotten from himself in five decades.

He tried something. That week, every time his bad mood started, he said to himself, out loud if he was alone, "This is my old brain doing what my old brain does. My hands do not know how to do this yet." It sounded silly at first. It sounded less silly by week three. By month two, the bad moods had not disappeared. But they were shorter. They were less lonely. And he was no longer beating himself up inside them, which had been half the weight all along.

What this means for you: You may not need a new technique. You may need a new framing. Treating yourself the way you would treat a child learning something hard is often more effective than any intervention you can buy.

4.6 Why Self Blame Does Not Work

One of the most counterintuitive findings in psychology is this: blaming yourself for your problems does not help you solve them. It actually makes them worse.

When you blame yourself harshly for being anxious, you trigger the threat system, which produces more anxiety. When you blame yourself harshly for feeling depressed, you generate more shame, which deepens depression. When you blame yourself harshly for not being more disciplined, you erode the exact sense of self-trust that discipline is built on (Gilbert, 2009; Neff, 2003).

The research is consistent across disorders, across cultures, and across age groups. Self-compassion (the opposite of self-blame) is associated with better mental health outcomes, lower anxiety, lower depression, higher life satisfaction, and even better physical health markers (Zessin et al., 2015; MacBeth & Gumley, 2012).

This does not mean you should excuse yourself for everything and stop trying to grow. It means the growth happens faster when you stop attacking yourself for needing it.

Think of it like teaching a child to ride a bike. If every time the child falls, you yell at them for being clumsy and stupid, the child learns slower, rides more cautiously, and often gives up. If every time the child falls, you say, "That is what falling looks like. Let us try again," the child learns faster and keeps going longer. The science on adult learning is remarkably similar. Shame is a poor teacher. Compassion is a better one.

You are the child in this analogy, and you are also the adult. Your job is to notice when the old self-blaming voice fires up and to gently, repeatedly, offer the other one.

4.7 When It Doesn't Work

Some readers hear the "not your fault, your responsibility" frame and their mind immediately does a strange thing. It uses the idea against them. The critic says, "Oh great, so now not only am I broken, but I am responsible for fixing it, and I am still not fixing it, so that is one more thing I am failing at."

If this happens to you, please notice what the critic did. It took a helpful framework and turned it into another weapon. The framework itself was not the problem. The critic's reflex to find new weapons was the problem.

Three things to try:

1. When the critic does this, simply name it out loud. "The critic is trying to use this idea to attack me." Naming breaks the spell. The weapon becomes visible, and once it is visible, it has less power.

2. Read section 4.4 again, but this time read only the "not your fault" part. Sit with it for a few minutes. You do not need to action anything today. You do not need to fix yourself today. You are allowed to take in the relief before the work.

3. If the shame from reading this chapter has gotten heavier rather than lighter, pause for a few days. Some readers need time for the old frame to loosen before the new frame can land. That is normal and it is not a failure of reading.

If the critic has been with you for a long time, it will take more than one chapter to quiet. Expect that. Do not measure progress in hours. Measure it in months.

4.8 The Main Ideas

Your brain is the product of a long evolutionary history, and it is not perfectly suited to the life you are living today. It was built to watch for danger, remember threats, stay close to the group, and react fast. In modern life, those ancient systems often fire without a real target, which produces anxiety, self-criticism, and shame that feel personal but are actually deeply human.

The single most important reframe in this chapter is the two-part sentence: your brain is not your fault, and your brain is your responsibility. Both halves matter. Dropping either one collapses the whole idea.

Self-blame is not the engine of change. Self-compassion is. This is counterintuitive for most of us, because we have been told our whole lives that being hard on ourselves is how we grow. The research is clear, and the opposite is true. People who treat themselves the way they would treat a struggling child learn faster, recover quicker, and stay with hard things longer.

This chapter was the philosophical foundation of everything that comes next. The chapters ahead will get more concrete. They will introduce you to the three emotional systems that live inside you, and they will start to show you how to work with them. The work is practical. But the work only lands if the framing is right.

Nothing is wrong with you. You are human. And being human, as it turns out, is a very specific thing, with very specific instructions that no one ever handed you at birth.

In the next chapter, you will meet the three circles.

Chapter 5: The Three Circles Inside You

Yuki sat on her kitchen floor at 7:14 p.m. on a Wednesday, eating cold leftover rice straight out of the container with her fingers. She had not planned to be on the kitchen floor. An hour ago, she had been answering emails at her dining table. Thirty minutes ago, she had been pacing around her living room. Ten minutes ago, she had been crying in the bathroom. Now she was on the floor because the floor felt like the only surface that made sense.

She had not eaten all day. She had been running on coffee and the flood of stress hormones that had hit when her manager had pinged her at 9 a.m. with "do you have a minute to chat?" The chat had turned out to be about a minor scheduling question. But in the hours between the ping and the meeting, Yuki's body had been in full emergency mode. Her heart rate had been up. Her breath had been shallow. Her mind had been running worst-case scenarios on a loop.

After the meeting, instead of relaxing, she had flipped into overdrive. She had plowed through her task list at double speed, replying to every email, opening every tab, saying yes to every request, all while a little voice in her head kept saying *you have to make up for this, you have to prove you are fine, do more, move faster.* By 6 p.m., she had run out of tasks, and the crash hit.

Now she was on the floor, eating rice, exhausted in a way that felt too big for one day.

Three different systems had been running her, all day, in rotation. She just did not have names for them yet.

What You'll Get From This Chapter

This chapter introduces the single most useful model in all of CFT: the three circles. You will learn about the threat system, the drive system, and the soothing system, what each one does, what each one feels like in your body, and why the goal is balance, not silence. By the end, you will have a framework that, once it is in your head, will change how you understand almost every emotional experience you have from here on out. Most readers say this chapter is the one they come back to most often.

5.1 Meet The Three Systems

Paul Gilbert, drawing on decades of research in affective neuroscience, describes three main emotion regulation systems that every human has (Gilbert, 2009; Depue & Morrone-Strupinsky, 2005). He calls them the threat system, the drive system, and the soothing system. Many people find it helpful to picture them as three overlapping circles, each with its own color.

Red is the threat system. Its job is protection. It handles fear, anger, anxiety, and disgust. It pulls your hand off the hot pan, makes you flinch at loud noises, and keeps you alert when you sense something is off. When red is running, your body is fast, tight, and watchful.

Blue is the drive system. Its job is resource-seeking. It gives you motivation, excitement, pleasure, and the push to chase goals, status, achievement, and reward. When blue is running, your body is energized, focused, and forward-leaning.

Green is the soothing system. Its job is safeness and connection. It handles contentment, calm, affection, and the sense of being cared for. When green is running, your body is settled, warm, and open.

All three systems are necessary. None of them is bad. The threat system kept your ancestors alive. The drive system helped them find food, mates, and status. The soothing system allowed them to rest, to bond with their children, and to trust their tribe. You need all three, because life requires all three.

The trouble comes when the systems fall out of balance. Most of the people who find their way to a book like this one are running high in red, high in blue, and low in green. That combination is exhausting, and it is what was happening to Yuki on her kitchen floor.

5.2 The Threat System

The threat system is the oldest, fastest, and most dominant of the three. Evolution gave it priority for a simple reason: missing a threat once could kill you, while missing a reward once was usually fine. Your ancestors were descended from the humans who treated every rustle in the grass as a lion. The humans who assumed it was nothing got eaten.

You inherited that priority. Your threat system is always online, always scanning, and always ready to override the other two. When it fires, you feel it first in the body, before you even know what is happening.

The threat system delivers three main emotion types: fear, anger, and disgust. Each has its own flavor, but they share a common tone of urgency and discomfort. You might feel: A racing heart, fast shallow breathing, muscle tension, A sudden urge to run, fight, or freeze, Hyper-alertness, scanning for what is wrong, Tight focus on the threatening thing, and narrow thinking, A body that feels hot, cold, or jittery, and A mind that keeps looping back to the same worry.

When red is running, your thinking changes too. You become more negative, more pessimistic, and more prone to catastrophic predictions. This is not a flaw. It is the threat system's built-in bias. It is better (evolutionarily speaking) to assume the worst and be wrong than to assume the best and get eaten.

Modern life triggers the threat system constantly, and often for things that are not actual threats. A curt email from your boss. A neighbor's raised voice. A notification with a red dot. A thought about the future. Your threat system does not know these things are not lions. It just knows you flinched, and it takes over.

5.3 The Drive System

The drive system is the engine that gets you out of bed, makes you want things, and pushes you to pursue them. It is the system that lights up when you are excited about a new project, chasing a goal, earning a reward, or winning something. When it is running well, you feel motivated, focused, and alive.

The drive system runs on dopamine, largely, and it is designed to reward the act of pursuit even more than the act of achievement. This is part of why the anticipation of a reward often feels better than the reward itself. It is also why people get caught in endless loops of chasing the next thing, because the chase is the payoff (Depue & Morrone-Strupinsky, 2005).

When blue is running healthily, it looks like: Engagement with work or projects, Enthusiasm for new experiences, Setting goals and pursuing them, The pleasure of achievement and progress, and A sense of momentum and forward movement.

When blue runs out of balance, it looks like: Compulsive productivity, unable to stop or rest, Feeling empty when a goal is reached, and immediately needing the next, Using busyness to avoid other emotions, Addiction patterns with substances, food, work, phones, shopping, and Burnout, where the engine overheats and seizes.

A lot of high-achieving readers of this book live mostly in blue. They are successful by external measures. They are exhausted internally. The drive system was never meant to run at full speed all day, every day. It was meant to pulse. Pursue, achieve, rest, pursue again.

Yuki's afternoon was a blue-system blowout. When she came out of her manager's meeting, instead of letting her body settle, she pushed into drive. She used task completion as a way to feel in control. It worked for about four hours. Then the engine ran out of fuel and she ended up on the floor.

5.4 A Real Example

Miguel is forty-two, an entrepreneur, on his second startup. He spent his twenties and thirties proving himself. He built companies. He sold one for decent money. He exercises. He reads. He has a partner he loves. On paper, he has all the pieces of a good life.

In practice, he has not felt a moment of contentment in five years.

His pattern is a familiar one. Every morning, he wakes up already running. He checks his phone before his feet hit the floor. He drinks coffee while reviewing his task list. He pushes through the day with a constant low-grade urgency, as if something is always about to go wrong. On weekends, he plans hikes, projects, and workouts, because sitting still feels unbearable. When he hits a business milestone, he feels a small flicker of satisfaction that lasts about ninety seconds before he starts thinking about the next milestone.

What he tried first was meditation. He downloaded three different apps. He did ten-minute sessions every morning for about six weeks. He reports that he "got better at meditating" but felt no actual peace. He gave up.

What eventually helped was a conversation with his partner, who said, gently, over breakfast, "Love, you are wired. All the time. You have been wired for years. Your body does not know how to be off."

That sentence unlocked something. Miguel started reading about nervous system regulation. He came across the three circles model. He realized, with something close to shock, that he had been living almost entirely in red and blue for his entire adult life. Red (the constant low-grade urgency) and blue (the constant task completion). His green circle was so underdeveloped he could not even identify what it would feel like to live there.

He did not solve his pattern in a week. He is still working on it. But he started doing something small. Once a day, for five minutes, he sat on a chair by his window and drank a cup of tea. He did not check his phone. He did not plan the next thing. He just sat. The first few times, he said, he nearly climbed out of his own skin. By week four, he started to feel something he had not felt in years. A softness. A quiet.

He did not know the word for it at the time. It was green, showing up for the first time in a long time.

What this means for you: If you cannot even imagine what the soothing system feels like, that is information. It means you have been running in red and blue for so long that green has atrophied. It has not disappeared. It just needs practice.

5.5 The Soothing System

The soothing system is the one most underdeveloped in readers of this book. It is also the one that changes everything once it starts to grow.

The soothing system is your built-in calm. It is the system that lets you feel safe without needing to achieve anything. It is the system that produces the feeling of being held by someone who loves you, the relief of coming home after a hard day, the contentment of a quiet morning with nothing demanded of you. It runs on different brain chemistry than red or blue. Oxytocin and endogenous opioids are involved. The parasympathetic nervous system is engaged. Your heart rate slows. Your breathing deepens. Your body softens (Porges, 2007; Carter, 1998).

When green is running, you might feel: A sense of warmth in the chest or belly, Slow, deep, easy breathing, Loose shoulders, relaxed jaw, A feeling of being settled, grounded, or at home, A softness in the face and around the eyes, and A quiet mind, without the urgency of threat or the pull of drive.

The soothing system is linked, in evolution, to caregiving and being cared for. It is the system that develops most strongly in children who received consistent, warm caregiving, and that often does not develop well in children who did not. This is a hard sentence. Read it once, breathe, and keep going.

If you grew up in a household where care was inconsistent, critical, frightening, absent, or conditional, your green circle probably did not get the input it needed to grow strong. That is not your fault. It does mean the work ahead might feel harder for you than for someone whose green system was nourished early. It also means the work is more important, not less.

The soothing system can be grown at any age. The science is clear on this. Compassion-based practices, slow breathing, warm physical contact, safe relationships, and time in nature all strengthen it (Kok et al., 2013; Kirby et al., 2017). Every practice in Part Four of this book is designed to feed your green circle.

5.6 Another Real Example

Layla is twenty-nine. Her early childhood was chaotic. Her mother was loving but unpredictable. Her father was not around. She grew up constantly scanning for her mother's mood, learning how to be small, quiet, and helpful. By the time she was an adult, she had a very loud red circle, a very active blue circle (she worked too much, dated too intensely, and exercised to the point of injury), and almost no green circle at all.

She went to therapy at twenty-seven. Her therapist asked her, during the second session, "When was the last time you felt safe?"

Layla could not answer. Not because she could not think of an example. Because the question felt incomprehensible. Safe from what? She had a good apartment. She had a stable job. She was not in any physical danger. What did the therapist mean by safe?

The therapist tried again. "When was the last time you felt like you could let your guard down?"

Silence. Longer. Then Layla said, very quietly, "I do not know if I have ever let my guard down."

That answer became the center of her work. Not solving it. Just knowing it. For months, she worked on small doses of green. Warm baths. One trusted friend. A weighted blanket. Mornings where she did not check her phone. Her therapist taught her soothing rhythm breathing (a practice you will meet in Chapter 11.0 of this book). She did it badly. She kept doing it.

Eighteen months in, Layla had a moment. She was sitting on her couch on a Sunday afternoon, reading a novel. Her cat was curled up against her leg. Afternoon sun was coming through the window. She noticed something she had never noticed before. Her shoulders were not around her ears. Her jaw was not clenched. Her chest felt warm. She was not thinking about anything. She was just there.

It lasted maybe four minutes. She started crying, gently, when she realized what it was. It was safe. It was green. It had arrived, not as a breakthrough, but as a quiet Sunday afternoon.

What this means for you: The soothing system does not announce itself. It does not arrive as a revelation. It shows up as a Sunday afternoon where your shoulders are down and you are not thinking about anything. The work is to notice these moments when they happen, and slowly, patiently, to build more of them.

5.7 Balance, Not Silence

One common misreading of the three circles model is that the goal is to silence red and blue and live only in green. That is not the goal. That would not be healthy. That would not even be possible.

You need your threat system. It keeps you safe. You need your drive system. It gets you through your day, pays your bills, and builds your life. You need your soothing system. It lets you rest, connect, and recover.

The goal of CFT is balance. It is about being able to move between the three systems appropriately, depending on what the situation calls for. Red when there is an actual threat. Blue when there is a goal worth pursuing. Green when it is time to rest, connect, or simply be. Most readers of this book can find red and blue in their sleep. They need to grow green, not to replace the others, but to give the others somewhere to land when they finish their work.

A useful way to picture a healthy mind: the three circles overlap and share space. One might be more active at any given moment, depending on the demands of life, but none of them is stuck on or stuck off. When the threat fires, it does its job, and then the soothing system helps the body come down. When drive pushes you toward a goal, it does its work, and then soothing lets you rest before the next push.

If your green circle is weak, red has nowhere to land when it finishes firing. So red stays on. Drive has no off-switch, so drive keeps running. You end up on a kitchen floor at 7:14 p.m. eating rice with your fingers.

The work of this book is not to make red or blue go away. It is to build the green that lets them rest.

5.8 When It Doesn't Work

Some readers read this chapter and feel a wave of grief. They realize, often for the first time, how rarely they have experienced the soothing system. The grief can be heavy. It is also, usually, a sign that the model has landed.

Other readers read this chapter and try to immediately go into green. They sit down, try to relax, and find that their body will not cooperate. They feel worse, not better. They conclude they are failing at the model.

Both responses are common. Here is what to do.

If grief comes up, let it. Do not try to fix it today. Grief is what happens when you finally have language for something you have been missing for years. It is its own kind of recognition. Put the book down for a day or two. Let the grief move through. It will usually soften.

If you try to activate green and cannot, that is also normal. Three things to try:

1. Do not aim for green directly. Aim for small drops of it. A warm drink. A hand on your chest. A slow exhale. Two minutes, not twenty.

2. Notice when green shows up on its own, even briefly. A moment of warmth when you see a pet. A moment of rest when you sit down. Your job is not to manufacture green; it is to notice the green you already have.

3. Accept that red will probably fire while you are trying to do green. That is not failure. That is information. Your threat system does not trust softness yet. It will, with time.

If this chapter has stirred up something large (grief, trauma memories, a sense of hopelessness), please set the book aside and talk to a therapist. This model is a foundation, but some foundations need human company to land safely.

5.9 The Shape Of Your Week

Before we move on, try one small thing this week. You do not have to do it right. You just have to do it.

For seven days, at the end of each day, take about two minutes. Ask yourself three questions.

1. When was red running today? Where did I feel it? 2. When was blue running today? Was it healthy drive or frantic drive? 3. Was there any moment of green? Even a few seconds?

You are not trying to change anything. You are just noticing. Most readers discover, over a week, that they spend the majority of their day in red, a significant chunk in blue, and very little in green. That is not a failure. That is your starting map. You cannot change a pattern you have not seen.

The next chapter takes you deeper into what happens when red runs the whole show.

5.10 Pulling It Together

You have three emotion regulation systems. Red is threat, for protection. Blue is drive, for pursuit. Green is soothing, for safeness and connection. All three are needed. All three have value. The goal is balance.

Most people who struggle with self-criticism, shame, anxiety, or burnout are running heavy in red and blue and light in green. Their threat systems fire too easily and will not settle. Their drive systems run without an off-switch. Their soothing systems were underfed, often in childhood, and have not had a chance to grow.

None of this is a failure of character. It is a reflection of biology, environment, and history. It is also workable. The soothing system can be strengthened at any age. Every practice in the second half of this book is designed to do exactly that.

For the next week, notice which circle is running at any given moment. Do not try to change it. Just name it. "This is red. This is blue. This is green." The naming itself begins to shift things, because naming puts a little space between you and the system you are in. In that space, choice becomes possible.

In the next chapter, we look at what happens when red takes over completely, and why the critic and the worrier both live there.

Chapter 6: When Threat Takes Over

Omar was in line at the grocery store. A regular Tuesday evening. He had a basket with eggs, bread, coffee, and a bag of apples. The woman in front of him was taking a long time. The cashier was new and kept looking confused. Omar glanced at the clock on his phone. He had a video call in forty minutes. Plenty of time. He knew he had plenty of time.

His body did not agree.

His heart started pounding. His chest got tight. His face got hot. He felt a wave of impatience that surprised him with its sharpness. He caught himself glaring at the back of the woman's head. He had a thought that went something like, *who raised her, why does she not just move, why is this cashier incompetent.* Even as the thought formed, another part of him watched it happen and felt ashamed. These were not thoughts he held. He did not actually believe these things. He was not an impatient man in general.

But he was also, in that moment, exactly an impatient man. His body was in full threat activation over nothing at all. Over a slow checkout line.

By the time he got to his car, his heart was still pounding. He sat with his hand on the wheel for a minute. He did not drive yet. He just sat there, realizing something he had realized many times before and never quite absorbed. His nervous system had just run an entire emergency sequence for absolutely no reason. And it was going to do it again later tonight, probably, and tomorrow, and the day after that, and he did not know how to make it stop.

What You'll Get From This Chapter

This chapter takes you deeper into the red circle. You will learn how the threat system hijacks your body, your thinking, and your behavior, often in situations that do not call for it. You will see why the inner critic and the chronic worrier both live in this system. You will get a clearer picture of what threat actually does to you, so that in later chapters, when you start doing practices to settle it, you will understand what you are trying to settle.

6.1 How Threat Hijacks You

The threat system is fast. That is its main feature. It evolved to get you out of harm's way before your conscious mind could weigh options. By the time your thinking brain has registered that something is happening, your threat system has already triggered a cascade of physical changes (LeDoux, 1996).

Here is what happens, roughly, when your threat system fires:

Your amygdala, a small almond-shaped structure deep in the brain, detects a potential threat. It does not wait for confirmation. It sends a signal to the hypothalamus. The hypothalamus triggers the release of adrenaline and cortisol. Your heart rate goes up. Your breathing gets faster and shallower. Blood flow shifts from the digestive system to the large muscles, because if this is a real threat, you might need to run or fight. Your pupils dilate. Your palms sweat. Your mouth gets dry. Your hearing sharpens.

All of this happens in under a second. Your conscious mind catches up a few seconds later. By the time you are even aware that you are anxious, the physiological event has been in motion for a while.

This cascade is incredibly useful if there is actually a tiger. It is less useful if you are standing in line at a grocery store. The system cannot tell the difference. It just fires.

Once the threat system is fully activated, your thinking also changes. You become more focused on the threat, less able to see the bigger picture, and more prone to catastrophic predictions. Research shows that under high threat activation, creative problem-solving drops significantly, working memory narrows, and the capacity to take in new information shrinks (McEwen, 2007). You are, in effect, dumber in the service of being faster. For a real tiger, that is a good trade. For a slow cashier, it is not.

6.2 The Body Knows First

One of the most important things to understand about the threat system is that it lives in the body, not in your thoughts. By the time you are thinking anxious thoughts, your body has already been anxious for a while. The thoughts are downstream of the physiology, not the other way around.

This is why thinking your way out of anxiety often does not work. By the time you try to reason with yourself, your body has already flipped into red. Your reasoning brain is operating on a system that is flooded with stress hormones. Under those conditions, reasoning has limited power.

Common physical signs that your threat system is running: Heart rate faster than the situation warrants, Breathing shallow, high in the chest, or holding your breath, Tightness in the jaw, shoulders, neck, or chest, A knot or fluttering in the stomach, Sweating, cold hands, or a dry mouth, Restlessness, the urge to move, fidget, or pace, Frozen stillness, as if you cannot move, and Sudden fatigue or collapse.

If you learn to notice these body signs early, you can intervene before your mind gets fully swept up. Many readers discover that they have been running in threat mode for years without realizing it, because the signs have become so familiar they feel like baseline.

This is part of why the practices later in this book emphasize the body. Soothing rhythm breathing. Grounding through posture. Safe place imagery. These are not random exercises. They are body-first interventions on a body-first problem. You cannot talk the threat system down. You have to breathe it down, posture it down, imagine it down.

6.3 A Real Example

Isabella is thirty-six, a physician. She has been a doctor for ten years. She is good at her job. Patients like her. Her reviews are strong.

Every Monday morning, from about 5 a.m. to 7:30 a.m., she is in full threat activation. Her heart pounds. She has trouble breathing. She feels nauseous. She replays cases from the previous week, worries about the patients she will see that day, and mentally rehearses conversations she might have to have. By the time she gets to the hospital, she is already exhausted.

She has been doing this for most of her career. She has tried beta blockers. She has tried running in the morning. She has tried meditation. The Monday morning surge keeps happening. She has come to accept it as part of the cost of her job.

What shifted things was not a new intervention. It was a conversation with her sister-in-law, who mentioned in passing that she had started working with a therapist who talked about the nervous system. Her sister-in-law said, "My therapist says that what I was calling anxiety is actually my body being stuck in on-mode."

Something about that phrase, stuck in on-mode, hit Isabella. She realized that her Monday mornings were not about the upcoming work. They were her threat system firing because her threat system had learned to fire on Monday mornings. The trigger was no longer the actual patients or cases. The trigger was Monday itself, her body's conditioned expectation that something bad was about to happen.

What she tried was something almost absurdly simple. On Sunday night, she started doing three minutes of slow breathing before bed. Four counts in, six counts out. She did not try to do it for twenty minutes. She did not try to meditate. She just slowed her breath for three minutes. She did the same thing when she woke up Monday morning, before she got out of bed.

The first week, nothing changed. The second week, her Monday was slightly less awful. By month three, her Monday morning surge had dropped to about thirty percent of what it had been. Not gone. But manageable. The physician in her noted that three minutes of slow breathing, twice a day, had done more than any medication she had ever tried.

What this means for you: The threat system is not just responding to real-time threats. It is also responding to learned patterns. Once your body has learned to fire in a certain situation, it will keep firing, even after the actual danger is gone. The way out is not to think differently. The way out is to give the body new signals, repeatedly, over weeks and months.

6.4 The Thinking Traps Of Threat

When red is running, your thinking tilts in specific directions. Cognitive therapists have catalogued these tilts extensively (Beck & Haigh, 2014). A short tour of the main ones:

Catastrophizing. Your mind jumps to the worst possible outcome. Your boss wants to talk to you, so you are about to be fired. Your friend has not replied to a text in two hours, so they are angry at you. Every small signal points to a catastrophe that is not actually likely.

Mind reading. Your mind decides you know what other people are thinking, and what they are thinking is usually bad. They are judging you. They are annoyed. They think you are incompetent. There is rarely any evidence. The threat system does not need evidence. It needs certainty, and it manufactures it.

All or nothing thinking. Situations become black or white. You are either succeeding or failing. You are either loved or rejected. The grey zones, which is where most of life actually lives, disappear under threat.

Should statements. You flood yourself with should, must, and have to. *I should be over this by now. I should not feel this way. I must get this right.* Each should is a small attack on the self for failing to be different from what you currently are.

Personalization. You take responsibility for things that are not your responsibility. A coworker is quiet, so it must be something you did. A meeting went badly, so it must be your fault. The threat system does this because making you the cause is how it tries to give you control. If the problem is you, then maybe you can fix it. The logic is flawed, but the threat system is not interested in good logic.

Filtering. Your mind zooms in on whatever is wrong and cannot see what is right. A presentation gets ten positive comments and one critical one. The critical one is the only one you remember. This is not a character flaw. It is threat-system attention. It is pulling focus to the potential danger.

You do not need to memorize this list. Noticing even one of these patterns in your own thinking, in real time, is enough. The naming creates space. Once you can see that your mind is catastrophizing, you have room to breathe.

6.5 Another Real Example

Lin, forty-four, is a freelance graphic designer. She lives with an inner critic and a chronic worry habit that have been with her since childhood.

Her worry pattern looks like this. She wakes up around 4 a.m. and her mind starts reviewing. Finances. A client who has been slow to respond. A health concern she has been putting off. Her mother's declining memory. Her daughter's grades. Each topic gets about three minutes of spinning, then her mind jumps to the next. By 5 a.m. she is exhausted. By 6 a.m. she has given up on sleeping and is out of bed, already anxious, already tired, already preparing for a day that has not even started.

What she tried first was the thing most of us try. She tried to think her way out. She would argue with the worries. *My finances are actually fine. The client will probably respond. The health thing is probably nothing.* The arguments worked for about ninety seconds before her mind found a new worry, or the same worry in a new outfit. She called it whack-a-mole. The moles always won.

What helped her was a frame change. Her therapist explained the three circles. Her therapist said something like, "When you wake up at 4 a.m., your body is already in red. The worry is not causing the anxiety. The anxiety is generating the worry. Your threat system needs something to chew on, so your mind serves it up topics."

Lin had never thought of it that way. She had always assumed the worries came first and the body followed. Once she understood the order, she stopped trying to argue with the worries. She started treating 4 a.m. as a body problem, not a thinking problem. She kept a heating pad by the bed. When she woke up, she put it on her stomach. She did slow breathing. She did not try to solve the worries. She just tried to give her body a signal that it was not, in fact, in danger.

The worries did not stop. They did get quieter. More importantly, she stopped fighting them, which meant she stopped getting more wound up by the fight itself. Some nights she went back to sleep. Some nights she read a novel until 5:30. Either way, she was not in combat with her own mind for two hours every morning.

What this means for you: Worry is often a downstream symptom of threat, not the cause of it. If your body is already in red, your mind will find topics to worry about. Treating the body first, and the topics second, is often the more effective order.

6.6 The Critic Lives Here

Here is the connection you need to remember. The inner critic you met in Chapter 1.0 lives in the threat system. Self-criticism is a red-circle behavior.

This is one of the most important ideas in CFT, and it takes most readers some time to fully absorb. The critic is not a neutral judge. The critic is a threat strategy. It beats you up in an attempt to keep you safe from external threat, by getting you to perform better, avoid mistakes, or pre-empt rejection by rejecting yourself first (Gilbert, 2000; Gilbert & Procter, 2006).

Once you see that the critic is part of your threat system, two things change. First, you stop trying to argue with it using logic, because threat-system behaviors do not respond well to logic. Second, you start to recognize that the critic will be loudest when your threat system is most activated. Hard days, bad sleep, financial stress, a fight with a partner, these are the days the critic will roar. It is not roaring because something new is wrong with you. It is roaring because your body is in red.

This has a practical implication. If you want to quiet your critic over time, the fastest route is not to argue with it. The fastest route is to lower overall threat activation. When your body feels safer, the critic gets quieter. The critic is running on fuel. Reduce the fuel, reduce the fire.

This does not mean you ignore the critic. It means you recognize that the critic is a symptom of a system that is running too hot, and you work on the system. The rest of this book is largely about how to do that.

6.7 When It Doesn't Work

Some readers try to notice their threat system firing and cannot find it. They do not feel their heart pounding. They do not notice the tight chest. They just feel, in their words, "like this is just how I am."

This is very common, especially for people who have been in threat mode for years. The signs get so familiar they become invisible. You cannot notice your shoulders being up because your shoulders have been up for as long as you can remember. The body's alarm has faded into what feels like a neutral baseline.

Three things to try:

1. Check in with your body several times a day, at the same times (for example, every time you wash your hands, or every time you start the car). Just ask, "Where is my breath? Where is my tension?" You are not trying to fix anything. You are building a map.

2. Notice the moments after. You may not be able to catch the threat system firing, but you can often catch the aftermath. The exhaustion after a conversation. The sudden appetite for something sweet. The urge to lie down. These are often threat-system residue. Use them as clues.

3. Ask one person who knows you well what they notice about you. Say something like, "How can you tell when I am stressed?" They probably know better than you do. The external view is sometimes the only one available when you have lost the internal one.

If you feel, after reading this chapter, that you have been in threat mode for years and you do not know how to get out, please know that the rest of this book is aimed exactly at this problem. You are not too far gone. The nervous system is plastic. It responds to consistent, small inputs over time. You do not need to fix everything this week. You need to start, gently.

6.8 Before You Move On

Your threat system is old, fast, and powerful. It evolved to protect you, and it still does, often. It also fires in situations that do not need it, which is where most of your anxiety, irritability, and self-criticism come from.

Threat is a body event first and a thinking event second. By the time you catch your anxious thoughts, your physiology has already been going for a while. This is why body-based practices (breathing, posture, imagery, slow movement) tend to do more than thought-based arguments with yourself. The body came first. The body needs to be addressed first.

Your inner critic lives in your threat system. It is not a neutral judge. It is a protection strategy that no longer serves you. The way to quiet it is not to argue with it. The way is to lower overall threat activation in the body, so the critic has less fuel to run on.

In the next chapter, you will meet the soothing system in more detail. You will learn why it is often weak, what it feels like when it is strong, and what you can begin to do to grow it. That chapter is the doorway into Part Four, where the actual practices live. For now, you have finished the part of the book that names the problem and the structure. The next chapter is the first hint of the way out.

Chapter 7: Growing Your Soothing System

Nicole drove home from her first therapy session feeling strange. She was fifty-three. She had signed up for therapy because her adult daughter had told her, with love, that she was "the most tense person I have ever met." Nicole had laughed. Her daughter had not laughed back. Nicole had booked the appointment the next day.

The therapist had asked her, in that first session, a simple question. "What helps you feel calm?"

Nicole had opened her mouth to answer and realized she did not know. She said something about wine with dinner. The therapist nodded and asked, "Other than substances or numbing?"

Nicole tried again. She mentioned her dog. That one counted. Then she tried to think of other things, and could not, really. She mentioned vacations, but she always came back from vacations exhausted. She mentioned spa days, but she only had them once a year and she spent half of them worrying about her email. She mentioned reading, but her mind wandered. She mentioned hot baths, but she always rushed them.

The therapist wrote something down and said, "Okay. That is what we are going to work on."

On the drive home, Nicole realized she was fifty-three years old, and she had never seriously worked on the question of what made her feel safe and calm. She had worked on her career. She had worked on her marriage. She had worked on her parenting. She had worked on her weight. She had never worked on her own peace.

What You'll Get From This Chapter

This chapter is about the green circle, the soothing system that most readers of this book barely know. You will learn why it is so often weak, what it actually feels like when it is working, and how it can be grown at any age. This is the doorway into Part Four, where you will learn the practices that feed it. For now, your job is to understand the system, so that when you meet the practices, you will know what they are pointing at.

7.1 The System You Barely Know

The soothing system is not just relaxation. It is not just the absence of stress. It is a distinct physiological state, with its own hormones, its own neural circuits, and its own felt sense (Porges, 2011; Uvnäs-Moberg, 1998).

When the soothing system is running, your parasympathetic nervous system is engaged. Your heart rate slows. Your breathing becomes slow and full, reaching into your belly rather than staying up in your chest. Your blood pressure drops slightly. Your digestive system turns on. Your face softens. Your voice, if you speak, gets warmer and slower. Oxytocin rises, especially if there is physical contact or a sense of social connection. The fight-flight chemistry of the threat system recedes.

Crucially, the soothing system is linked in evolution to caregiving and being cared for. It developed in mammals who needed to bond with their offspring and with their social group. The signals that activate it are signals of safety, warmth, and connection. A parent's gentle voice. A soft touch. Eye contact that is kind. The smell of home. These signals are not incidental. They are what green runs on (Carter, 1998; Mikulincer & Shaver, 2007).

Many readers have never had a good felt sense of the soothing system. They have had brief tastes, often in moments they did not fully register at the time: a quiet afternoon, a loved pet, a specific song, a particular smell. These tastes were green. But if you did not know to name them, you may not have known to build more of them.

This matters because the soothing system, like any system, gets stronger with use and weaker with disuse. If your life has trained you to live mostly in red and blue, your green has atrophied. Not permanently. But it has lost capacity that can be rebuilt.

7.2 Why Green Is Often Weak

There are many reasons someone's soothing system might be underdeveloped. Three are worth knowing about, because they are common and because recognizing them can take the shame out of the experience.

Early caregiving. The soothing system develops most strongly in the first few years of life, through contact with caregivers who respond warmly, consistently, and with attunement. Children who receive this kind of caregiving build a strong internal sense of safeness that they carry forward. Children who do not, often do not (Mikulincer & Shaver, 2007). This is not a blame of parents; many parents were doing their best under hard conditions. It is simply a description of how the system develops. If your early caregiving was inconsistent, critical, frightening, absent, or conditional, your green circle did not get the input it needed.

Cultural and social context. Some cultures value hardness, striving, stoicism, and the suppression of softness. Boys and men in many parts of the world are explicitly discouraged from displaying or cultivating what green looks like. So are girls and women in certain professional settings. People from marginalized communities often learn early that softness is not safe, because the world has not treated their softness gently. These environmental messages can stay with you long after the environment has changed.

Trauma. If you experienced abuse, violence, or sustained danger at any point in your life, your threat system learned to stay on, and your soothing system learned that it was not safe to come online. The body remembered. Even when the danger is long over, the system can stay wired for threat. This is not a failure of willpower. It is a sensible adaptation to a situation that no longer exists.

If any of these apply to you, please know that your green circle not being strong is not evidence of anything wrong with you. It is evidence of a life where the conditions for green were hard to come by. The work ahead is not to fix a defect. It is to provide, now, what was not provided then.

7.3 A Real Example

Akira is forty-seven. He grew up in a household where showing emotion was not acceptable. His father was a man of few words, most of them critical. His mother was anxious and easily overwhelmed, so Akira learned early to manage his own feelings to avoid burdening her. By the time he was an adult, he did not know how to be soothed. He had never really experienced it.

He was successful. He had a good marriage. His wife loved him. She would, sometimes, reach out to touch his shoulder when he looked stressed, and he would flinch. He did not mean to. His body just did it. He would apologize, she would smile sadly, and the moment would pass.

His turning point came in his forties, when he got a puppy for his daughter. The puppy, a small mutt from a shelter, was nervous and shy. She would not come out from under the couch for the first week. Akira spent hours lying on the floor next to the couch, not reaching for her, just being there. Eventually she came out. Eventually she let him touch her. Eventually, months later, she would crawl into his lap and fall asleep there, her warm body pressed against his chest.

He noticed, one evening, that when the dog was sleeping on him, his body did something it had never done before. His shoulders dropped. His breathing slowed. He felt warm in a way that did not come from any blanket. He felt, in a word he would not have used out loud, safe.

He started sitting with the dog deliberately. Twenty minutes at a time. He was not trying to meditate. He was not trying to fix himself. He was just noticing what was happening in his body while the dog was on him.

Over the course of about a year, his body began to generalize. He started to feel small versions of that same green feeling in other places. With his wife, when she sat next to him on the couch. With his daughter, when she told him a long story over dinner. With a friend, when they walked together through a park. The dog had taught his body something that forty-seven years of life had not. His nervous system had learned a new setting.

What this means for you: You may not need a technique to grow your green circle. You may need an experience. A safe being. A trusted presence. A body that allows itself to be near another body without flinching. Animals often do this for people. So do trusted humans. So, eventually, can you for yourself, but often the first teacher is another being.

7.4 How The Body Soothes Itself

The soothing system is something your body does. It is not something you think. This distinction matters, because if you try to reason yourself into green, you will fail, and conclude something is wrong with you. Nothing is wrong with you. You are just using the wrong tool.

The body has several built-in paths to the soothing system. Once you know them, you can start using them deliberately. These are not random self-help tips. They map onto the actual physiology of the parasympathetic nervous system and the vagus nerve (Porges, 2007).

Slow, full breathing, especially long exhales. When you exhale longer than you inhale, you signal the vagus nerve to activate the parasympathetic system. Four counts in, six counts out, is a common starting ratio. This is the physiological basis of soothing rhythm breathing, which you will meet in Chapter 11.0.

Gentle warm touch. A hand on the chest. A hand over the heart. Both hands holding each other. Warm skin-to-skin contact releases oxytocin, which calms the threat system and activates the soothing system. This is why a hand on your own chest can feel surprisingly powerful. Your body does not know the difference, neurochemically, between your own warm hand and someone else's.

Safe eye contact with a trusted being. A pet, a loved person, sometimes even a photo. Kind eyes looking back at you signal safety to the oldest parts of the brain. The eyes of a predator do the opposite.

A warm environment. A warm bath. A weighted blanket. Warm drinks held in your hands. Warmth is not incidental. The body associates warmth with the safety of being near other bodies, which is one of the original signals of safeness.

Slow, gentle movement. Walking slowly. Stretching. Rocking. Anything that moves the body without stressing it. Fast or intense exercise activates drive. Slow, easy movement activates soothing.

Soft sounds. A trusted voice. Music that does not demand attention. The rustle of trees. White noise. Soft sounds signal that the environment is not dangerous.

Nature. Time in green spaces has been shown, in multiple studies, to lower cortisol, slow heart rate, and activate the parasympathetic system (Hartig et al., 2014). This is not a hippie idea. It is a physiology finding.

You do not have to do all of these. Most people find that two or three work well for them. Your job, over the next few weeks, is to experiment and find out which ones open the door for you.

7.5 Another Real Example

Aisha is thirty-one. She is a social worker. She has spent her whole career helping other people regulate their nervous systems, and she had no idea that her own was chronically in the red.

She figured it out, oddly, while waiting for a bus. She was on her way home from a particularly heavy day. A small boy was sitting with his mother at the bus stop. The mother was holding him. The boy was maybe three. He was fussy. The mother started humming, very softly, and stroking his back in slow circles. Within about two minutes, the boy's whole body had changed. His shoulders dropped. His eyes half-closed. He melted into her.

Aisha watched, and felt something she had not expected. A sharp pang of something close to longing. Not for her own mother, who had been overworked and emotionally unavailable. For what that boy was getting. For a body that knew how to let another body regulate it.

She had never known that. She had never melted into anyone. She had never, not as an adult, allowed her body to be soothed by someone else. She prided herself on her independence. She did not ask for help. She did not let her partner hold her when she was upset. She would pat her partner's shoulder and say "I am fine" and walk into the other room.

That bus stop moment changed something. She went home and, for the first time in her life, she asked her partner to just hold her. No problem to solve. No conversation. Just to hold. She cried for about twenty minutes. She had no idea she had so much inside. She was not crying about anything specific. Her body was releasing years of never being soothed.

Over the next year, she practiced receiving. She let her partner hug her without explaining. She asked for backrubs. She sat with her friend in silence instead of always talking. She took warm baths and actually stayed in them. She went for slow walks without a podcast. Small things. Daily things. Green-circle things.

She describes it as "relearning how to be human." She was not broken before. She was under-nourished. She had been feeding her drive system and her threat system for thirty years, and her soothing system had been starving. Now, she was feeding it. Slowly. A little every day.

What this means for you: Growing the soothing system is not dramatic. It is a series of small, daily acts of letting your body be nourished by safe input. Warm touch. Slow movement. Safe presence. Kind eyes. These are not extras. They are actual food for a system that might have been on a long fast.

7.6 What Growing It Feels Like

One question readers ask often: what will I notice as my soothing system strengthens? Here are some of the signs.

Your body settles faster after stress. Something upsetting happens, and you used to spiral for three days. Now you spiral for half a day. A conflict used to take a week to recover from. Now it takes an afternoon. The threat system still fires, but the soothing system catches up faster.

You notice softer moments you used to miss. The way sunlight comes through a window. A stranger smiling at you in a coffee shop. The feel of warm water on your hands. Small instances of green become visible, because you now have the sensitivity to register them.

You stop flinching at care. When someone offers you warmth, a compliment, a hug, a kind word, you receive it instead of deflecting. This one can be hard to notice at first, because the deflection happens automatically. Your partner or a friend may notice it before you do.

Your self-talk softens. Not because you are forcing it. Because the threat system is running less hot, and the critic, which lives in threat, has less fuel. You catch yourself being kinder, without having to try.

You can be alone with yourself. This one surprises people. When the soothing system is strong, solitude stops feeling like exposure and starts feeling like rest. You can sit in a room with no input, no phone, no task, and just be.

Small moments of rest feel possible. A five-minute pause does not send you into anxiety. A weekend without plans does not feel like a void. Rest stops being a threat.

These changes do not happen overnight. They happen in weeks and months, often unevenly. You might have a very good week and then a bad week. That is normal. The overall direction, over time, is toward more of these signs and fewer of the old ones. You are not meant to become a different person. You are meant to become a more nourished version of the person you already are.

7.7 When It Doesn't Work

Some readers try everything in this chapter and cannot feel green. Their body does not settle. Their shoulders do not drop. Slow breathing makes them more anxious, not less. Safe touch makes them want to flee.

If this is you, please listen carefully. You are not doing it wrong. You are describing one of the most common patterns in people with complex trauma histories, and it has a name in CFT. It is called fear of compassion. It is the nervous system learning, from early experience, that softness is unsafe. When someone offers care, the body expects the other shoe to drop. When you try to offer care to yourself, the body braces.

Three things to try:

1. Start smaller than you think you need to. A single slow breath. Not three minutes of slow breathing. One breath. Notice what happens. If nothing happens, that is still information. Try again tomorrow.

2. Pair soothing input with safety signals you trust. If your dog has always felt safe, do your slow breathing with your hand on the dog. If a specific room feels safer than others, practice there. You are not cheating. You are giving your system more support than it has had before.

3. Consider working with a therapist trained in trauma-informed CFT, somatic experiencing, or EMDR. Some nervous systems need human company to get into green for the first time, because the original injury happened in the context of another human. Books can introduce the ideas. Sometimes a body needs a body.

There is no shame in this. There is no prize for doing it alone. Some of the readers who have most benefited from CFT did the foundational green work in a therapist's office, and then continued it at home. The point is not the route. The point is that green grows.

7.8 The Short Answer

You have a soothing system. It may be weak. It was probably underfed for most of your life, for reasons that are not your fault. It can be grown at any age, through consistent, small inputs that your body recognizes as safety.

The soothing system is not something you think. It is something your body does. The paths into it are body-first: slow breathing with longer exhales, warm touch, safe eye contact, gentle movement, warmth, soft sounds, and time in nature. These are not random self-help tips. They are the actual physiological routes to the parasympathetic nervous system and the vagus nerve.

Growing green does not feel dramatic. It feels like a few fewer minutes of spiraling after a hard conversation. A softer self-talk that you did not consciously produce. A moment of warmth when you see a pet. A surprising capacity to sit still without panicking. You will not wake up one day as a new person. You will, over time, wake up as the person you have been with the old alarms turned down.

This chapter marks the end of Part Two. You now have the framework of the three circles, and you know why the work ahead focuses so heavily on the body. Part Three, the next three chapters, is about what compassion actually is, and why it is not soft, weak, or selfish. Part Four, after that, is where the practices live.

You have done the theoretical work. The practical work begins soon. For this week, simply notice. Where is red? Where is blue? Where is green? Do not try to change anything yet. Just see. The seeing is the first act of the work.

PART III: WHAT COMPASSION ACTUALLY IS

Chapter 8: Compassion Is Not Weakness

Mary had just won the biggest case of her career. Seven-figure settlement. The opposing counsel had conceded at the last possible moment, after nine months of grinding depositions and late nights. Her managing partner had pulled her aside in the hallway and said, "That was a beautiful piece of work." Her colleagues had cheered. Her inbox was full of congratulations.

At 10 p.m. that night, she was crying in her parked car in the garage under her building, and she did not know why.

She had driven home and stopped one level below her apartment and just sat. The tears came hard for about twenty minutes. When they slowed, she caught her reflection in the rearview mirror. Eye makeup destroyed. Face blotchy. She looked smaller than she felt.

Her phone buzzed. Her sister Zara was calling to congratulate her. Mary ignored it. She did not want to be warm with anyone right now. She did not want to be soft. Softness felt like a door she could not afford to open, because if she opened it, she was not sure she could close it again.

Mary had built her whole career on a specific kind of hardness. She had learned, from her first year at law school, that the people who made it were the ones who did not flinch. She had modeled herself on senior partners who worked ninety-hour weeks and spoke in clipped sentences. She had come to believe that kindness toward herself was a luxury she could not afford. If she eased off, she would lose her edge. Her edge was the thing that had gotten her here.

So she sat in the garage and refused to answer her sister. She would go upstairs, splash water on her face, have a glass of wine, and be ready for tomorrow. What she did not yet know was that the hardness she had built was the thing that had just broken her, silently, after the biggest win of her life. And that the research she had dismissed as soft was about to become the only thing that worked.

What You'll Get From This Chapter

This chapter dismantles the biggest misconception that keeps readers from trying CFT in the first place: that being kind to yourself will make you weak, lazy, or mediocre. You will learn why compassion is one of the most demanding human capacities, not the easiest. You will see the ten common fears that almost everyone has about self-compassion, and you will see the research showing that compassion-trained people actually achieve more, not less.

8.1 The Biggest Misconception

If you have made it to this chapter, congratulations on getting past the first real obstacle most readers face. Many people close CFT books in the introduction, or somewhere in the first part, because they hit a wall. The wall is this: somewhere, deep inside, they believe that being kinder to themselves will make them fail.

They believe, in no particular order, that self-compassion will make them: Lazy, Soft, Weak, Arrogant, Selfish, Mediocre, Vulnerable to being hurt by others, A pushover, Less motivated, and Stuck.

These beliefs are not stupid. They come from somewhere. Most of them were taught, directly or indirectly, by families, schools, workplaces, and cultures that rewarded hardness and punished softness. If you grew up in a competitive household, an immigrant family, a military family, a high-achieving profession, or any environment where self-criticism was framed as the engine of success, you inherited this frame. You are not dumb for holding it. You are well-trained.

The frame is also wrong in an important way. Research on self-compassion does not support the idea that kindness toward yourself makes you lazy or complacent. Instead, self-compassion is associated with better emotional resilience, healthier motivation, and less anxiety and depression (Neff, 2003; MacBeth & Gumley, 2012).

But research studies are not what will convince you. Your body needs a different kind of evidence. It needs to see, through lived experience, that warmth does not collapse you. That will take time. For now, a reframe will help.

8.2 The Firefighter Truth

Here is the reframe. Think about a firefighter running into a burning building to pull out a child.

What qualities does that firefighter have? List them in your head for a moment.

Most people say some combination of: brave, strong, skilled, committed, calm under pressure, focused, caring. Almost no one says: soft, lazy, weak, or self-indulgent.

Now notice what the firefighter is doing. They are being compassionate. They are sensitive to the child's suffering (the first part of compassion) and they have the courage, training, and strength to act on that sensitivity (the second part). Compassion is not the absence of strength. Compassion is strength applied in a specific direction.

Gilbert uses this example repeatedly, and readers find it disarming, because it punctures the myth in about thirty seconds

(Gilbert, 2009). Compassion is not sitting in a meadow being gentle with a butterfly. Compassion is running into hard places and doing hard things because they matter. The firefighter is one of the most intensely compassionate roles we have, and almost no one confuses a firefighter with a pushover.

The same thing applies to self-compassion. Being kind to yourself when you are suffering is not soft. Sitting with your own pain instead of running from it is not weak. Committing to the slow, hard work of changing long-standing patterns is not easy. These are some of the most demanding things a human can do. The critic, by contrast, is the easy path. Attacking yourself is quick. It feels like action. It takes almost no courage, because you already know the attack will work.

Real self-compassion takes more strength than self-criticism, not less.

8.3 A Real Example

Jennifer is forty-eight, a senior executive at a tech company. She has been on the self-criticism path her whole adult life. When her therapist suggested, in month three, that she try writing a kind letter to herself, Jennifer almost walked out. She said, out loud, "That is ridiculous. I did not get here by being nice to myself."

Her therapist, who had heard this before, simply asked, "Is what you are doing working?"

Jennifer paused. She had come to therapy because she was on her second antidepressant, could not sleep, had lost twenty pounds she did not need to lose, and had started crying in her car on the way to meetings. She did not answer out loud. But she took the assignment.

She did not like the letter she wrote. It felt fake. It felt like something a weaker person would write. She gave the exercise about twenty minutes and put it down.

Her therapist asked her to do it once a week for a month. Jennifer agreed grudgingly. By the fourth letter, something had shifted. She had started writing the letters as if she were writing to a younger colleague she cared about, someone she would never speak harshly to. The tone came more easily when she borrowed someone else's voice.

Six months later, Jennifer sent her therapist a one-line email. It said, "I am running harder than I ever have and I am not eating myself alive to do it." Her results at work had not declined. In some measurable ways, her results had improved. She was no longer burning out between quarters. She was no longer crying in her car. The critic still showed up. She just did not give it the whole microphone anymore.

What this means for you: You do not have to believe self-compassion will work. You can hold the skepticism and do the practice anyway. The evidence of how it works for you will come from your own experience, not from being convinced first.

8.4 The Ten Fears That Stop People

Dr. Chris Irons, who has worked with Gilbert for years, has written about the ten most common fears people carry about self-compassion. You may recognize several. Read through them and notice which ones feel true for you. Noticing them is the first step toward loosening their hold (Gilbert et al., 2011; Irons, 2019).

1. **If I am kind to myself, I will become lazy.** The fear that the critic is the only thing keeping you moving. 2. **Self-compassion is weak.** The belief that softness equals inability. 3. **I**

do not deserve it. The sense that something in your past or your nature makes you unworthy of kindness. 4. **If I let my guard down, something bad will happen.** The sense that softness is dangerous, often linked to trauma. 5. **Compassion will overwhelm me with sadness.** The fear that if you open the door to warmth, grief will flood in. 6. **I will become arrogant or selfish.** The confusion of compassion with self-indulgence. 7. **Others will judge me.** The fear that being kind to yourself will look bad to people who value hardness. 8. **My standards will drop.** The concern that without the critic, you will settle for less. 9. **It feels foreign.** The sense that compassion is for other people, not people like you. 10. **It will not work anyway.** The cynicism that says you have tried and it did not help.

Most readers resonate with three or four of these. A few resonate with all ten. Either way, the fears are predictable, treatable, and not evidence that you are doing anything wrong. The fears are part of the pattern the book was designed to address. Every practice ahead is, in some way, aimed at softening the fears, one by one, through direct experience.

8.5 Another Real Example

Wei is thirty-three, in recovery from alcohol use for about two years. Early in recovery, his sponsor kept using the phrase "self-compassion." Wei hated it. He thought it sounded like an excuse for bad behavior. He had spent his drinking years being "kind" to himself in ways that kept him sick. Another drink. Another pass. Another forgiveness he did not earn. The last thing he thought he needed was more of that.

His sponsor sat with him one night on a bench outside a meeting. He said, "What you were doing was not self-compassion. That was self-indulgence. They are opposites."

Wei did not understand at first. His sponsor tried an analogy. "Self-indulgence is giving a sick person what they want. Self-compassion is giving a sick person what they need, even when what they need is hard." Self-indulgence had been Wei drinking whenever he hurt, because drinking felt better. Self-compassion, his sponsor suggested, would have been Wei noticing that he was hurting and asking what would actually help. Most of the time, the answer would have been: not another drink.

That reframe changed something for Wei. He started to see self-compassion as the harder path, not the easier one. Going to the meeting when he did not want to. Calling his sponsor when shame told him to hide. Eating dinner when he wanted to skip it. Going to bed at a reasonable hour when his impulse was to stay up, scrolling, avoiding. These small, unglamorous acts were self-compassion. The drinking had been the opposite.

He still has hard days. But he no longer confuses what hurts him with what helps him. And his relapse prevention, he says, rests on this distinction more than on any other single idea he has encountered.

What this means for you: Self-compassion is not self-indulgence. They look similar from a distance. They are opposite in mechanism and in outcome. Self-compassion asks what you actually need. Self-indulgence asks what feels good right now, even if it harms you. If you have been confusing them, you are in good company, and the distinction will change how you see the rest of this book.

8.6 What The Research Actually Shows

The evidence on self-compassion has built steadily for over two decades. A short summary of what it says.

People higher in self-compassion: Experience less depression and anxiety (MacBeth & Gumley, 2012), Have better emotional regulation and bounce back faster from setbacks (Neff, 2003), Pursue personal goals with more persistence, not less (Terry & Leary, 2011), Take more responsibility for mistakes, not less, Have healthier relationships and are better partners, Report higher life satisfaction and wellbeing, Show better physical health markers, including lower inflammation and better sleep, and Are less likely to burn out in high-demand jobs.

The research does not support the idea that self-compassionate people are lazy, arrogant, or uncommitted. If you have been holding the belief that kindness toward yourself will lead to failure, the broader evidence points the other way, with self-compassion tending to track better wellbeing and more adaptive functioning (Zessin et al., 2015; Kirby et al., 2017).

This does not mean the belief will drop away because you read a paragraph. Beliefs installed by years of life experience take more than facts to shift. But you can now hold two things at once: the old belief that softness will ruin you, and the new knowledge that the research says otherwise. Over time, as you build practical experience, the research will slowly become the more trusted voice.

8.7 When It Doesn't Work

Some readers finish this chapter and notice their critic get louder. The critic does not like being named. It often responds to being seen by attacking harder, the way a bully escalates when finally confronted. Things to watch for: "Oh great, so now I am failing at compassion too.", "This book is for other people. I am actually different.", and "If I try this and it does not work, that will be more evidence that I am broken.".

If any of these arrive, that is normal. It does not mean the chapter has failed. It means the critic is defending its territory. Three things to try:

1. Name the critic's voice when it shows up. "The critic is trying to turn this book into another weapon." Naming works. It takes the voice out of first person and into third. 2. Do not try to argue with the resistance. Arguing feeds it. Just keep reading. Let the ideas sit. The practices in Part Four will do more than any argument can. 3. If you notice strong feelings coming up (grief, anger, a desire to throw the book), let them come. These are often signs that the content is landing somewhere real. Put the book down for a day. Come back.

If the resistance is overwhelming, it may help to talk to a therapist. Some fears of self-compassion are rooted in trauma and need more than a book to hold them.

8.8 The Quick Version

The single biggest obstacle to CFT is the belief that being kind to yourself will make you weak, lazy, or mediocre. Almost every reader carries this belief in some form. It is not stupid. It was taught. And it is wrong.

Compassion, done well, is one of the most demanding human capacities. The firefighter is the right image. Compassion is sensitivity to suffering plus the courage and skill to act on it. Self-compassion is not giving yourself a pass. It is taking your own suffering seriously and responding with wisdom, strength, and care. It is harder than self-criticism, not easier.

Ten common fears stand in the way, from "I will become lazy" to "I do not deserve it." You may recognize several. The fears are common and workable. They soften with practice, not with argument.

The research is clear. Self-compassionate people are not less motivated. They are more resilient, more persistent, and often healthier than their self-critical peers. Your own experience, not the research, will eventually be what convinces you. But you can start with the research and let your experience catch up.

In the next chapter, you will meet the two sides of compassion in more detail, and you will start to see that compassion has a shape. It is not a feeling. It is a skill. Skills can be learned.

Chapter 9: The Two Sides Of Kindness

Ananya got a call from her best friend at 11:47 p.m. on a Thursday. Her friend's father had died an hour earlier. The phone had been ringing in the silence of Ananya's dark bedroom, and she had known, before she picked up, what it was going to be.

She did pick up. Her friend was not crying yet. She was in that strange post-shock state where the sentences come out flat and logical. "My dad died. The nurse just called. I am driving there now."

Ananya said the thing she had rehearsed, somewhere inside herself, for exactly this kind of call. "I am so sorry. I am on my way. I will meet you at the hospital."

She did not hesitate. She got up. She put on clothes. She drove forty minutes through empty streets. She sat with her friend in a hospital waiting room for three hours. She held her friend's hand. She did not say the wrong thing. She did not try to fix it. She did not say, "At least he lived a long life," or any of the other sentences people say because they do not know what else to do. She just sat. When her friend cried, Ananya cried quietly alongside her. When her friend laughed, inappropriately, about a memory of her father ordering soup in a diner, Ananya laughed with her.

On the drive home the next morning, Ananya thought something odd. She had been able to do all of that for her friend. She had known, instinctively, what her friend needed. She had been present and kind and strong without effort. And yet, for her own self, she had no idea how to offer the same thing. When her own pain showed up, she turned away from it. When her own grief came, she buried it. When her own failures happened, she attacked herself. She had a warehouse of compassion for the people she loved. Her own door was locked from the inside.

What You'll Get From This Chapter

This chapter introduces the two sides of compassion and the three directions it can flow. You will learn that compassion is not a single thing but a pair of abilities that work together. You will see the six qualities that, together, make up a compassionate response. And you will find out which direction of compassion is hardest for you, because for most readers, one flow is much harder than the other two.

9.1 The Two Psychologies Of Compassion

Gilbert breaks compassion into two halves, which he calls the two psychologies. They are simple to describe and important to get right (Gilbert, 2010).

The first psychology is sensitivity to suffering. This is the capacity to notice that pain is happening, to turn toward it rather than away, and to allow yourself to feel it. It is the ability to stay present with something hard instead of flinching, numbing, distracting, or fleeing. When Ananya answered the phone and did not try to fix her friend's grief, she was exercising this first psychology. She was letting the suffering be what it was, without rushing to cover it.

The second psychology is the commitment to relieve or prevent suffering. This is the willingness to do something about it. Not to fix everything. Not to make the pain disappear. But to take wise action on behalf of the person suffering, including yourself. When Ananya got in her car and drove to the hospital, she was exercising this second psychology. She was not just feeling her friend's pain from a distance. She was moving toward it.

Both halves are necessary. Sensitivity without commitment is sympathy without help. You feel bad for the person but do nothing. Commitment without sensitivity is fix-it mode. You take action but miss what the person actually needs. Real compassion holds both, at once, in a wise balance.

This is where most attempts at self-compassion go wrong. People try one half. They try to be kind in their heads (sensitivity) without taking any actual action in their lives (commitment). Or they try to take action (commitment) without first acknowledging that they are suffering (sensitivity). Neither works alone. The two halves need each other.

9.2 The Six Qualities You Will Grow

Gilbert and others have broken the compassionate mind into six qualities that work together. These are not tests you pass or fail. They are muscles you build. You can be strong in some and weak in others, and the specific profile will shape the kind of work that will help you most (Gilbert, 2009).

Care for wellbeing. The underlying motivation to reduce suffering and support flourishing. This is the why of compassion. Without it, the other five do not fire.

Sensitivity. The ability to notice when suffering is present, in yourself or in others. This is what many self-critical people have turned off about themselves. They can see pain in others instantly. Their own pain is invisible to them until it becomes a crisis.

Sympathy. The capacity to be moved by what you notice. Not to stay neutral or distant. To let the suffering touch you. Sympathy is often confused with pity or weakness. It is actually an act of allowing yourself to be affected, which is a form of strength.

Distress tolerance. The ability to stay with hard feelings without flipping into avoidance, rage, or collapse. This is the quality that lets you sit with pain long enough to respond wisely. Without it, the compassionate impulse gets flooded by your own discomfort.

Empathy. The capacity to understand, from the inside, what someone is experiencing. Empathy is not the same as taking it on or losing yourself in it. Good empathy is knowing what it feels like without drowning in it.

Non-judgment. The willingness to notice suffering without immediately blaming someone for it, including yourself. This is the hardest one for self-critical people. Their first response to their own pain is often judgment about why they are in pain. Non-judgment loosens that reflex.

Read through the list again and notice which ones come easily and which ones are underdeveloped. Most readers of this book have reasonable sensitivity for others and almost none for themselves. Most have sympathy for others and contempt for themselves. Most have empathy for others and brutal judgment for themselves. The asymmetry is the pattern this book is trying to address.

9.3 A Real Example

Javier is fifty-six, a pediatrician. Over three decades of practice, he has sat with hundreds of parents whose children were sick, dying, or newly diagnosed with serious conditions. His colleagues describe him as exceptional at difficult conversations. Parents who have lost children still send him holiday cards fifteen years later. He is, by any reasonable measure, one of the most compassionate humans in his field.

His own son, when he was sixteen, was diagnosed with the same condition Javier had been treating in other children for twenty-five years. For the first week after the diagnosis, Javier was a wreck. He could not sleep. He could not eat. He snapped at his wife, which he rarely did. He found himself reviewing the chart obsessively, looking for things the specialists had missed, unable to trust colleagues he had trusted with other families for decades.

What was happening was not a failure of his compassion. It was the opposite. He had plenty of compassion. He could not direct it at himself. All his life, he had given it outward. He had built a whole career on the first flow, compassion to others. He had never learned to receive it from anyone, or to offer it to himself. When his own life became the thing that needed compassion, he had no practiced pathway.

His wife pointed this out to him, carefully, about two weeks in. She said, "Javier, if I were one of your parents right now, you would be so gentle with me. You are being so hard on yourself." He had not noticed. Once he noticed, he cried. He had been treating his own anguish as if it were a weakness to solve, not a suffering to be met with the same warmth he had offered a thousand other families.

He started doing one small thing. When his mind went hard on him, he said to himself, almost out loud: "If this were one of my patient families, what would I say?" The answer came easily, because the pathway was already paved for others. He just had to redirect the traffic.

What this means for you: You probably have a lot of compassion. It may be aimed almost entirely outward. The skill you are learning in this book is not how to manufacture compassion. It is how to redirect the compassion you already have, so that some of it flows toward you.

9.4 The Three Flows

Compassion can flow in three directions, and most people are strong in one, weak in another, and somewhere in the middle on the third (Gilbert, 2009).

Flow one: compassion to others. The ability to feel care for other people and act on it. This is the flow most humans find easiest, because it is the one most built into our social nature. Parents feel this for their children. Friends feel it for friends. Most people can access this flow, even if they are not warm by temperament, at least in specific circumstances.

Flow two: compassion from others. The ability to receive care when it is offered. To let a hug land. To hear a compliment without deflecting. To accept help without feeling indebted. This flow is where many readers stumble. They can give, but they cannot receive, because receiving requires vulnerability.

Flow three: compassion to self. The ability to direct warmth toward yourself when you are suffering. To treat yourself with the kindness you would offer a friend. To speak to yourself without contempt. This is usually the hardest flow for readers of this book, and it is the one CFT is most concerned with.

Each flow reinforces the others. If you have never received compassion from others, you will find it hard to give to yourself, because you have no internal model of what being cared for feels like. If you cannot give compassion to yourself, your compassion for others often becomes depleted, because you are giving from an empty well. If you give to others but cannot receive, you eventually burn out.

The practices in Part Four are designed to work all three flows. Soothing rhythm breathing and safe place imagery strengthen the self-flow directly. The compassionate other practice teaches you to receive, by imagining a figure who offers care you can let in. Compassionate letter writing lets you practice giving to yourself in a slow, deliberate way. Over time, the three flows come into better balance, and each one makes the others stronger.

9.5 Another Real Example

Amanda, forty-one, has always been the caretaker in her family. She is the one who organizes her parents' medical appointments, who picks up her sister's kids from school when needed, who checks in on her friends after breakups. She describes herself as "a giver."

What Amanda has never been able to do is ask for anything. When her husband offers to cook dinner, she says she is fine. When her friends ask how she is, she says good, even when she is not. When her mother offers to help with childcare, Amanda refuses. The receiving flow is almost completely shut down.

She went to a retreat last year where the teacher asked everyone to pair up and receive compassion from the other person for three minutes. The partner would simply sit across from Amanda and silently wish her wellbeing.

Amanda could not do it. She started to cry about thirty seconds in. Not because she was moved. Because she felt exposed. Her partner was looking at her with kindness, and her body did not know where to put it. She felt like she was taking something she had not earned.

Later that week, the teacher asked her why receiving was so hard. Amanda said, "If I let them in, I do not know how to say thank you enough. I am afraid I will not be able to repay it."

The teacher smiled gently and said, "What if you do not need to repay it?"

That sentence took Amanda six months to absorb. She had organized her entire adult life around earning care by giving care. The idea that she could receive without an immediate ledger balance felt almost impossible. She is still working on it. What has helped most is a small practice her teacher gave her. When someone offers her something, instead of deflecting, she says three words: "That is kind." That is all. She does not explain. She does not refuse. She does not promise to reciprocate. She just lets it land.

She reports that those three words are among the hardest she has ever learned to say.

What this means for you: Receiving is often harder than giving, especially for people who grew up earning love. The practice is not grand. It is letting one compliment land without deflecting. One offer of help accepted without explaining. These small acts begin to open a flow that has been shut for a long time.

9.6 Finding Your Blocked Flow

Take a moment with three questions. You do not need to write the answers down. Just notice.

First, think of a friend or family member you care about who is struggling. How easily can you feel compassion for them? Most readers find this flow reasonably available, even on a hard day. This is your outward flow.

Second, think of the last time someone offered you unconditional care. A hug. A compliment. A genuine "how are you?" without agenda. How did your body respond? Did you let it in, or did you deflect, minimize, or squirm? This is your incoming flow.

Third, think of the last time you made a real mistake or failed at something that mattered. How did you speak to yourself? Was your tone the same tone you would have used with the friend in question one? Or was it harsher, colder, more contemptuous? This is your inward flow.

Most readers of this book find that the outward flow is available, the incoming flow is uncomfortable, and the inward flow is almost non-existent. Once you see this pattern, you have a clear target. The work is to strengthen the flows that are weaker, slowly, over weeks and months.

9.7 When It Doesn't Work

Some readers try the three-flow exercise and cannot access any of them. They think of a loved one and feel nothing. They imagine receiving care and feel uncomfortable. They think of being kind to themselves and go blank.

This is not failure. This is a sign that your threat system is running high enough that compassion, in any direction, is temporarily offline. The body does not generate warmth when it is busy scanning for danger.

Three things to try:

1. Do not try to force the flows. Instead, go back to something simple. Three slow breaths. A hand on your chest. A minute of warm water on your hands. Ground the body first. The flows will become available when the threat system settles. 2. Notice if you can access compassion for a being that feels safer than a human. A pet. A tree you love. A child you know. Sometimes the outward flow opens first for non-human beings, because they are less complicated. 3. Try again in a few days, when you are less

depleted. Compassion has a physiological cost. You cannot access it when you are running on empty.

If you notice that the inward flow is not just blocked but actively frightening, please be gentle. Fear of self-compassion has deep roots. The rest of this book is built to help it loosen. You do not have to force anything this week.

9.8 Closing Thoughts

Compassion is not one thing. It is two halves working together: sensitivity to suffering and the commitment to do something about it. Both halves are necessary. Sensitivity alone is paralysis. Action alone is fix-it mode. Real compassion holds both.

Compassion is made up of six qualities: care for wellbeing, sensitivity, sympathy, distress tolerance, empathy, and non-judgment. You can have these in abundance for others and none for yourself. That pattern is extremely common in readers of this book. It is workable. The asymmetry can be evened out over time.

Compassion flows in three directions: to others, from others, and to yourself. Each flow reinforces the others. Most readers of this book find the outward flow easiest, the incoming flow uncomfortable, and the inward flow nearly impossible. Knowing your pattern is the first step to rebalancing it.

This week, do one small experiment. When someone offers you kindness (a compliment, a hug, an offer of help), practice letting it land. Do not deflect. Do not explain. Just notice it and say something small like "thank you" or "that is kind." You do not need to perform receiving. You just need to stop actively stopping it.

In the next chapter, you will meet something CFT calls the compassionate self. You will be surprised to learn that it already lives inside you. Your job is to start listening to it.

Chapter 10: Meeting Your Compassionate Self

Ming sat on the floor of her closet with the door closed. It was 2 p.m. on a Wednesday. She had come home from work for her lunch break and had not been able to make herself go back. Her phone had been buzzing with messages for the last twenty minutes. She was not crying. She was just sitting, knees pulled up, back against the wall of hanging shirts.

Her daughter had called her that morning from college. Her daughter had been struggling. Anxiety. Not eating well. Not sleeping. Ming had listened. Ming had said the right things. Ming had reminded her daughter that she was loved, that her feelings made sense, that it was brave to ask for help, that this would pass. Her daughter had hung up feeling better.

Ming had hung up and gone into the closet.

The thing was, Ming had been feeling the same things as her daughter. For weeks. Maybe months. She had been anxious, not eating well, and not sleeping. The difference was that when she said those things to her daughter, she meant them. When she thought them about herself, she heard a different voice, one that said: you are fifty-three, you should have this figured out by now, stop being dramatic, go back to work.

What Ming could not yet see, sitting in the closet with her knees pulled up, was that the person she had been on the phone with her daughter was already inside her. The calm one. The kind one. The one who knew what to say. That person had not been invented for the call. That person had been there all along. Ming had just been listening to a different voice when it came to herself.

She did not need to become a kinder person. She needed to find the one she already had access to, and start letting that one speak, sometimes, inward.

What You'll Get From This Chapter

This chapter introduces what CFT calls the compassionate self. It is not a character you have to invent. It is a version of you that already lives inside, one you have probably accessed many times for other people. You will learn what its qualities are, why it can feel hard to reach for yourself, and how to begin building the practice of embodying it. This chapter contains the first full guided exercise of the book. You will learn a simple, grounded way to start meeting your compassionate self on a regular basis.

10.1 A Self You Already Have

The compassionate self is not a separate being. It is not a spirit. It is not something you have to earn. It is a set of qualities you already possess, which you have probably been expressing for other people for years, while assuming you did not have access to them.

Every reader of this book has, at some point, shown up for someone else in a compassionate way. You have comforted a friend. You have listened to a stranger. You have sat with a child who was scared. You have been patient with someone who was struggling. You have said the right thing when it mattered. Each of those moments was an expression of your compassionate self.

The question is not if you have a compassionate self. You do. The question is if you can direct it inward, toward your own suffering, with the same natural ease you direct it outward toward others.

Gilbert describes the compassionate self as having four core qualities, and these are the qualities you are learning to inhabit deliberately (Gilbert, 2010):

Wisdom. An understanding of how suffering actually works. The knowledge that life is hard, that your brain is tricky, that much of your pain is not your fault. Wisdom is what keeps compassion from sliding into pity or fix-it mode. The compassionate self knows what it is dealing with.

Strength. The capacity to stay grounded in the presence of difficult emotions. Not to collapse. Not to panic. Not to flee. The compassionate self is not a soft voice that disappears when things get hard. It is strong, rooted, steady.

Warmth. The felt quality of caring. Not theoretical. Not performed. A genuine warmth in the chest and the voice that signals: I am here for you. I care what happens to you.

Caring commitment. The willingness to take wise action to relieve suffering. Not just to feel bad that you are struggling, but to do something about it. The compassionate self is committed to your wellbeing, even when you are not.

These four qualities together are what you are building as you read this book. Each practice in Part Four strengthens one or more of them. Over time, the four qualities become more available, more integrated, and more automatic. They become less a performance and more a felt reality.

10.2 Why It Can Feel Hard To Reach

If you have access to these qualities when you offer them to others, why is it so hard to turn them toward yourself? There are several reasons, and understanding them will save you a lot of frustration.

You are not practiced. Skill with any capacity comes from use. If you have never directed compassion inward, the neural pathway for it is underdeveloped. This is not a character flaw. It is a wiring issue, and wiring changes with practice.

Your critic gets in the way. The moment you try to speak kindly to yourself, the critic often shows up to interrupt. "That sounds fake. You do not really deserve that. Stop being dramatic." The critic has been running the show for a long time. It does not give up the microphone easily.

Your body has learned to brace. If you grew up without consistent warmth, or if you experienced trauma, your body learned that softness was unsafe. When you try to turn warmth toward yourself, your body can interpret the kindness as a threat and contract. This is the backdraft phenomenon you will meet in Chapter 16.0.

You cannot see yourself clearly. Most people have an easier time feeling compassion for another person than for themselves, partly because they can see the other person from the outside. They can see the struggle, the effort, the suffering. From the inside, you see mostly your own failures and flaws. The perspective is broken.

The compassionate self practice is designed to address all four of these. It gives you a deliberate practice space, it gives you a position to speak from that is not the critic, it grounds the practice in the body, and it asks you to step outside yourself, imaginatively, so you can see yourself the way you would see a friend.

10.3 A Real Example

David is forty-four, a marriage and family therapist. He has been helping people regulate their emotions for fifteen years. He knows every technique in the book. When his teenage son was diagnosed with depression last year, David could not stop crying. It was not proportional, he told himself. He should be able to handle this. He did it every day at work.

Over several sessions with his own therapist, David discovered something strange. The voice he used with his clients was warm, patient, and steady. The voice in his head, directed at himself, was harsh, impatient, and dismissive. He had been operating with two completely different voices for years without noticing.

His therapist tried something. She asked David to close his eyes and imagine that he was sitting across from a younger version of himself, a version who was going through what he was going through now. She asked him to speak to that younger David the way he would speak to a client. David hesitated. Then he did it.

He said, out loud, sitting in his therapist's office, things like: "You are carrying a lot right now. It makes sense that you are struggling. Your son is going through something hard, and you love him, and watching someone you love suffer is one of the most painful human experiences. You are not failing. You are feeling. There is a difference."

He broke down halfway through. Not because he was making it up. Because he meant every word, and he had never, once, said any of those sentences to himself. He had been saying versions of those sentences to clients for fifteen years. He had never turned them inward.

That practice became the thing that worked for him. Twice a week, he would sit for ten minutes and talk to the younger version of himself, out loud or silently, from the voice he already used for other people. He described it as finally giving himself the same quality of care he had been giving away for years.

What this means for you: Your compassionate self already exists. It speaks in the voice you use with people you care about. The practice is to find that voice and aim it in a new direction. You are not inventing. You are redirecting.

10.4 Your First Practice

Here is a simple practice to begin meeting your compassionate self. You do not need to be good at it. You do not need to feel anything. You just need to try.

Find a quiet place. Sit upright in a chair, feet on the floor, hands resting on your thighs. Close your eyes or lower your gaze.

Take three slow breaths, breathing a little deeper than usual. Let your face soften. Let your shoulders drop.

Now imagine, as vividly as you can, that you are taking on the role of a deeply compassionate person. Think of this as putting on a costume. You do not have to be this person. You are playing the part.

Picture what this compassionate person is like. What is their posture? Steady, upright, grounded. What is their facial expression? Soft, warm, present. What is the tone of their voice? Calm, low, kind.

This compassionate person has four qualities. They have **wisdom**, which means they understand that suffering is part of being human. They have **strength**, which means they do not collapse when things get hard. They have **warmth**, which means they genuinely care. They have **commitment**, which means they take wise action on behalf of those they care for.

Spend a minute imagining yourself inhabiting each of these qualities. Feel what it would be like to sit with that posture. Feel what it would be like to breathe at that pace. Feel what it would be like to have a voice that steady and that warm.

Now, from this compassionate self, think of yourself as you were this morning. Not a younger version. Just you, today. Notice something that was hard about your day. Notice yourself, from the outside, the way a kind friend might.

And, from this compassionate self, say something to that version of you. It does not have to be profound. It could be: "Today was hard, and you kept going." Or: "You are carrying a lot, and I see it." Or: "I am here for you."

Stay for another minute. Then let the image fade, return to your normal breathing, and open your eyes.

That is the whole practice. It takes about five minutes. You do not have to do it well. You just have to do it.

10.5 Another Real Example

Zara is twenty-nine. When she tried this practice for the first time, nothing happened. She sat in her chair. She closed her eyes. She tried to imagine the compassionate self. She felt silly. She could not picture any of it clearly. She could not find a voice. She opened her eyes after about three minutes, sighed, and decided the practice was not for her.

Her therapist encouraged her to try again the next week. And the next. Zara did it, reluctantly, six times over six weeks. She felt nothing, every time.

On the seventh attempt, something shifted. It was not dramatic. She was sitting in her chair, doing the practice, when she caught a small glimpse of something. A feeling of slight warmth in her chest. A sense that the practice was not silly. A moment where the phrase she said to her morning self landed with a tiny amount of real meaning. She felt, for about four seconds, like she was actually there for herself.

The feeling faded. But it had been real. That was the beginning.

By month four, the practice was reliably producing something. Not big emotions. Just a settled quality, a sense of being in contact with a kinder part of herself. She started doing the practice on days when her critic had been loud, and she noticed that the critic was quieter for a few hours afterward. By month six, she could bring the compassionate self into difficult moments in real life. A tough email. A difficult conversation with a family member. A moment of self-judgment. She could, almost automatically now, step into the compassionate posture, soften her face, and ask herself what a kind response would look like.

She was not a different person. She had the same critic, the same history, the same struggles. What had changed was that the compassionate self, which had always been there, was now reachable. She had built the path.

What this means for you: The practice does not work in week one. Or week three. For many readers, it produces nothing for the first several attempts. That is normal. The practice is teaching your brain and body a new pathway, and pathways take repetition to form. If you do this practice once a week for eight weeks and still feel nothing, keep going. The learning is happening underneath the surface.

10.6 What To Expect

Here is what to expect over the next few months of working with the compassionate self practice, drawn from what readers and clients commonly report.

Weeks one to three. You will probably feel silly. The practice may seem fake. You may not feel anything. You may feel mildly irritated or bored. This is almost universal. Do not stop.

Weeks four to eight. Small moments begin to appear. A flicker of warmth. A sense of the posture starting to feel real. The voice you are trying to access begins to sound slightly less foreign. You may have one or two moments that genuinely move you.

Months three to six. The compassionate self becomes more reliable. You can access it in the practice setting fairly consistently. You begin to notice it arising spontaneously in daily life, sometimes without you calling it in.

Months six and beyond. The compassionate self becomes an integrated part of how you respond to your own life. It does not replace the critic. It lives alongside it. But it is now available as a real option when you need it.

Nothing about this timeline is rigid. Some readers move faster. Some move slower. What matters is not the speed. What matters is that you keep practicing, even when nothing seems to be happening. The nervous system is slow to change, and it changes through consistent, gentle repetition. Like any skill.

10.7 When It Doesn't Work

Some readers try the compassionate self practice and feel worse, not better. A few things can cause this.

If the practice brings up grief, that is usually a sign that something important is surfacing. Compassion can activate old pain, because it points at what was missing. Let the grief come. Do not push it away. It is part of the process.

If the practice triggers anxiety, your threat system may be interpreting the softness as a threat. This is particularly common for people with trauma histories. Three things to try:

1. Do the practice for only one minute, not five. Build up slowly. 2. Keep your eyes open, focused on a neutral object, rather than closed. Closed eyes can intensify the practice for some people. 3. Pair the practice with something physical that feels safe, like a hand on your chest or a weighted blanket. Physical grounding can make the imagery less destabilizing.

If the practice produces flooding (memories, intense emotions, dissociation), please stop and consider working with a therapist. Some people need professional support to do this work safely, especially if early caregiving was traumatic. There is no failure in needing help. The practice will still be available when you have the support to hold it.

10.8 Where You Are Now

You have reached the end of Part Three. You now know what compassion actually is. It is not softness. It is not weakness. It is a pair of capacities (sensitivity to suffering and the commitment to relieve it) that together make up one of the most demanding human skills. It has six qualities, three flows, and a clear structure you can learn.

You also know that your compassionate self is not something you have to invent. It already lives inside you. You have been expressing it for other people, probably for years. The work ahead is to redirect some of that compassion inward, so that the flow toward yourself becomes as available as the flow toward others.

You have done the first guided practice of the book. If it felt awkward, good. That means you actually tried it. If it felt powerful, good. That means the pathway is starting to open. If it felt nothing, good. That means you are at the beginning of a skill, and the skill is coming.

Part Four begins now. It is the part of the book where the actual practices live. Each chapter will teach one practice in depth, with step-by-step guidance, common difficulties, and guidance on what to do when it does not work. The first one you will meet is soothing rhythm breathing. It is the simplest and most important practice in all of CFT. It is also the one most readers skip, because it seems too basic to be worth doing. Please do not skip it. It is the foundation everything else is built on.

Turn the page when you are ready.

PART IV: YOUR FIRST PRACTICES

Chapter 11: Breathing Your Body Calm

Hassan had been lying in bed for forty minutes. He knew he was not going to fall asleep any time soon. His mind was running. His chest was tight. His heart was not racing, exactly, but it was up there, somewhere faster than it should be for 11:30 p.m. on a Tuesday.

He had been trying every trick he knew. He had counted backward from a hundred. He had imagined his favorite beach. He had done the mental body scan his yoga instructor had taught him, and gotten halfway through before his mind veered off. He had tried to think about nothing, which always works out as well as it sounds.

Finally, he gave up and just lay there. He breathed in. He breathed out. He was not trying to do anything. He was just breathing, because breathing is what he was already doing, and nothing else was working.

He noticed, without planning it, that his exhales were getting a little longer than his inhales. It happened on its own. In through the nose for a few seconds. Out through the mouth for a few more. His jaw loosened a little. His shoulders dropped about half an inch. His chest, which had been tight, became slightly less tight.

He stayed with that pattern. In. Out. A little longer on the out. After about five minutes, his heart had settled. After ten, he was yawning. He fell asleep still breathing that way.

The next morning, he realized something that felt almost too simple to be real. Of all the things he had tried, the one that had worked was the thing he was already doing. He had just slowed it down.

What You'll Get From This Chapter

This chapter teaches you the foundational practice of CFT: soothing rhythm breathing. It is the simplest of all the practices. It is also, for many readers, the one that produces the most change. You will learn why breathing works on a physiological level, how to do it, what posture and facial expression add to the practice, and what to do when your mind wanders, gets bored, or fights it. By the end, you will have a practice you can do in five minutes a day, in one minute in a crisis, and in thirty seconds almost anywhere.

11.1 Why Breath Changes Everything

Your breath is the one part of your nervous system you can consciously control that also directly affects the parts you cannot. Heart rate. Blood pressure. The balance between your sympathetic (fight or flight) and parasympathetic (rest and digest) systems. You cannot directly slow your heart by deciding to. You can slow your heart indirectly, reliably, by slowing and deepening your breath (Porges, 2007; Jerath et al., 2006).

The key lever is the vagus nerve. This is a long, wandering nerve that connects your brainstem to your heart, lungs, digestive system, and many other organs. It is the main highway of the parasympathetic nervous system. When it fires, your body calms down. Your heart rate slows. Your breathing deepens. Your digestive system activates. Your face softens. Your sense of threat decreases.

One of the fastest ways to activate the vagus nerve is through slow, deep breathing, especially breathing where the exhale is longer than the inhale. This is not a magic trick. It is a physiological mechanism that has been studied for decades. When you exhale slowly, the vagus nerve is stimulated, and your body shifts toward the soothing system. Every time. Even if your mind is still racing. Even if you feel nothing. The mechanism does not require your belief. It just requires the breath.

This is why breath is the foundation of almost every contemplative tradition. It is also why breath is the foundation of CFT. Gilbert built soothing rhythm breathing as the entry point to the whole approach, because everything else in the book requires a nervous system that is at least slightly settled. If your threat system is running at full volume, you cannot meaningfully engage the compassionate self, the safe place, or the compassionate other. You need the breath first.

11.2 Posture Matters Too

Breathing alone is powerful. Breathing combined with the right posture and facial expression is more powerful still. Your body is an integrated system. The signals you send through one channel reinforce the signals you send through others.

For soothing rhythm breathing, the posture is simple. Sit upright in a chair, feet flat on the floor, hands resting on your thighs. Imagine a string at the top of your head gently pulling you upward. Your spine is long, but not stiff. Your shoulders are relaxed. Your chest is open.

This posture is neither collapsed nor military. Collapse signals defeat to the body. Military rigidity signals vigilance. Upright and relaxed signals safety with dignity. Your body reads these signals constantly. Sitting well during the practice tells your body that you are present, grounded, and not in danger.

The facial expression is just as important. Allow a gentle, soft expression to settle on your face. Imagine a very small half-smile at the corners of your mouth. Not a grin. Not a performance. Just the faintest upward turn. Soften your forehead. Soften around your eyes. Unclench your jaw.

This matters more than it sounds. The muscles of your face are deeply connected to your emotional state, and the connection runs in both directions. Anxious feelings produce a tense face. A tense face produces more anxious feelings. By deliberately softening your face, you send a signal back to your body that the threat has passed. The body, which cannot distinguish between a real safety signal and a deliberate one, responds.

11.3 The Full Practice

Here is the practice, step by step. Read through once. Then try it. The first time will probably feel awkward. That is fine.

1. Find a quiet place where you will not be interrupted for five to ten minutes. Sit in a chair with your feet flat on the floor. Rest your hands on your thighs.

2. Lengthen your spine without straining. Let your shoulders drop. Let your jaw relax. Let your face soften into a very small half-smile.

3. Close your eyes or lower your gaze to a soft focus on the floor in front of you.

4. Notice your breath without changing it at first. Just notice where it is. Is it high in your chest? Low in your belly? Fast or slow?

5. Begin to slow and deepen your breath. Let the inhale come down into your belly. Feel your belly rise slightly on the in-breath and fall slightly on the out-breath.

6. Find a rhythm where your exhale is slightly longer than your inhale. A common starting pattern is four counts in through the

nose, a very brief pause, and six counts out through the mouth or nose. Find what feels natural for you. You do not have to count rigidly.

7. Continue this slow rhythm for five to ten minutes. If your mind wanders, simply return to the breath when you notice. No judgment. No self-criticism. Just return.

8. When you are ready to finish, take three normal breaths. Open your eyes. Notice how your body feels compared to when you started.

That is the whole practice. It is built to be simple on purpose. Simple practices, done consistently, change the nervous system more than complex practices done occasionally.

11.4 A Real Example

Aisha was one of the many readers who almost gave up on soothing rhythm breathing after the first week. She tried it on a Monday. She sat in her chair. She slowed her breath. She set a timer for five minutes. At minute two, she was already thinking about lunch. At minute three, she was thinking about a difficult email. At minute four, she was bored. By minute five, she concluded that the practice was not for her.

She told her therapist the next week, "I do not have the attention span for this. It is not working."

Her therapist asked her a simple question. "Did you do it?"

Aisha said yes, she had done it, but her mind had been all over the place.

Her therapist said, "That is the practice. The mind wandering and coming back, over and over, is not an interruption to the practice. It is the practice. You were doing it right."

Aisha had assumed, like many beginners, that a good session was one where her mind stayed still. In fact, a good session, her therapist explained, was one where she noticed her mind wandering and came back to the breath, again and again. Every return was a rep. Every rep strengthened the neural pathway. The wandering was not the failure. The returning was the work.

She went back to the practice with new eyes. She did it every day for two weeks. Some days she returned her attention to the breath thirty times in five minutes. Some days twice. She stopped keeping score. By the third week, she noticed something strange. Outside of the practice, in the middle of her workday, she caught herself slowing her breath automatically when she felt stressed. Her body had learned the rhythm. It had generalized.

What this means for you: The point of the practice is not to have a quiet mind. The point is to return, over and over, to the breath, when the mind wanders. Each return is the exercise, the way each push-up is the exercise at the gym. If you return one hundred times in five minutes, you have done one hundred reps. That is not failure. That is the practice working exactly as designed.

11.5 When Your Mind Wanders

Your mind will wander. This is not a problem. This is the nature of minds. The practice does not require you to have no thoughts. It requires you to notice when you have wandered and to come back, gently.

Three gentle things to try when you notice your mind has taken off:

First, do not get angry at yourself. The critic will show up. It will say, "You cannot even do this. Five minutes and you cannot focus for thirty seconds." Notice the voice. Name it. Do not argue. Just come back to the breath.

Second, use a simple word as an anchor. Some readers silently say "in" on the inhale and "out" on the exhale. Others say "soft" on the exhale. The word gives the mind something to hold, and when it wanders, the word is an easy place to return to.

Third, if the mind keeps wandering to the same topic, name the topic silently. "Thinking about work." "Thinking about my mother." "Thinking about what to have for dinner." Name it. Then return. The naming prevents the topic from grabbing you for ten minutes without you realizing it.

Over time, the gap between wandering and noticing gets shorter. In week one, you might be gone for two minutes before you realize. By month three, you might notice within five seconds. This is real progress. It is also invisible. You have to trust that the practice is doing its work even when you cannot see it.

11.6 Another Real Example

Ravi had been doing soothing rhythm breathing for about four months when he had his moment. He was at work, in a meeting that was going badly. A coworker was being unreasonable. Ravi could feel his chest getting tight. His jaw clenching. The old familiar spiral starting.

Without thinking about it, he took a slow breath in through his nose, and an even slower breath out through his mouth. Four seconds in. Six seconds out. He did it twice more. He did not leave the meeting. He did not announce the practice. He just breathed.

His body settled. Not all the way. But enough that he stayed present. Enough that he responded to his coworker with clarity rather than reactivity. After the meeting, he realized that four months of five-minutes-a-day practice had just paid off. His body had learned the rhythm. It was available now, even in a meeting, even under pressure, even without him deciding to use it.

This is what the practice builds, slowly, over months. Not just a dedicated quiet time. A skill the body can call up in the middle of life, without warning, without needing a chair or a closed door.

What this means for you: The real payoff of soothing rhythm breathing is not what you feel during the practice. It is what happens to your body during the rest of your day, as the slow-breath pathway becomes more accessible. You are not practicing to feel good for five minutes. You are practicing to have a different nervous system across your whole life.

11.7 Using It In Hard Moments

Once you have practiced for a few weeks, you will have access to a one-minute version and a thirty-second version that you can use almost anywhere.

The one-minute version. When you feel stress rising, pause. Sit upright. Soften your face. Breathe in slowly for a count of four. Breathe out slowly for a count of six. Do this for about six cycles, which will take roughly one minute. Return to what you were doing. Your body will be measurably calmer.

The thirty-second version. In a meeting. In a car. In line. When you feel the surge. Three slow breaths, each exhale deliberately slower than the inhale. Jaw soft. Shoulders down. Thirty seconds. You will not transform your whole state. You will interrupt the escalation. Often, that is enough.

These shorter versions only work if you have been doing the longer version regularly. The short versions draw on the pathway you have built in the dedicated practice. Without the dedicated practice, a thirty-second breath exercise in a stressful moment often does very little. With the practice in place, thirty seconds can reset the whole nervous system.

11.8 When It Doesn't Work

Some readers try soothing rhythm breathing and feel worse, not better. There are a few common causes.

If slowing your breath makes you feel anxious or short of breath, you may be trying too hard. Forced deep breathing can actually trigger the threat system in some people. Try starting with a gentler version. Just slow your breath a little. Do not try to fill your lungs completely. Let the breath be easy. Ease matters more than depth.

If the practice triggers intense emotions, that is often a sign that your body has been holding a lot of tension, and the slowing down is letting some of it move. This is usually a good thing, but it can be overwhelming. Three things to try:

1. Shorten the practice to two or three minutes, not ten. Slow expansion is better than flooding. 2. Keep your eyes open, focused on a neutral object, rather than closed. This keeps some of your attention in the external world. 3. Pair the practice with a warm drink, a weighted blanket, or some other physical grounding. The additional safety signals help the body tolerate the slowing.

If you have a trauma history, some breath practices can trigger flashbacks or dissociation. This is not uncommon and is not a failure. Consider working with a trauma-informed therapist who can modify the practice for your specific system. You can still benefit from this book. You may just need support to do this particular practice safely.

If nothing seems to happen at all, even after weeks, keep going. The body takes time. The pathway is forming even if you cannot feel it yet. Measure the results in what happens outside the practice, not inside it. Is there any moment during the day where your body settles a little faster after stress? Is there any moment where you breathe slowly without being told to? These are the signs. They are quiet. They are real.

11.9 One More Look

Soothing rhythm breathing is the foundation of CFT practice. It is not optional. Every other practice in this book depends on it. If you skip this chapter and try to go straight to the imagery or the letter writing, you will find those practices much harder to engage with, because your body will not be in the state they require.

The practice is simple. Slow the breath. Lengthen the exhale. Upright posture. Soft face. Five to ten minutes a day. Come back to the breath every time your mind wanders, without judgment. The returning is the practice.

The payoff is not always visible during the session. The payoff shows up in your life, in the ways your body responds to stress, in how quickly you recover from hard moments, in the unexpected slow breath that arrives in a meeting. You cannot force that payoff. You can only practice, consistently, and let the pathway form.

For this week, commit to five minutes a day for seven days. That is thirty-five minutes total. You can find thirty-five minutes. Do not try to do twenty minutes a day and fail by day three. Do five. Be boring about it. Let the consistency do the work.

In the next chapter, you will learn to build a safe place inside yourself. That practice builds directly on this one. Without the breath, the imagery has nowhere to land. With the breath, the imagery becomes real.

Chapter 12: Building A Safe Place Inside

Kenji was on a plane. Window seat. He was two hours into a four-hour flight. The turbulence had been bad for the last twenty minutes. Not dangerous. Just the kind of bumping that rattles the cart and makes the flight attendants sit down. The woman next to him was fine. The man across the aisle was reading. Kenji was not fine.

His heart was pounding. His palms were damp. He had the seatbelt gripped with both hands. He knew, with his thinking brain, that turbulence was normal. He flew often. He had been told, by multiple pilots, that turbulence could not take down a plane. None of that helped.

He had been trying to read. He could not focus. He had been trying to listen to music. The music felt like noise. He was doing the slow breathing he had been practicing for six weeks. It was helping a little. Not enough.

He closed his eyes. He tried something his therapist had taught him a month ago. He had practiced it at home. He had never tried it in the air.

He imagined his grandfather's back porch. The porch in a small town in the mountains, where he had spent summers as a child. The wooden railing, faded gray. The view of the valley. The sound of the creek below. The smell of pine. His grandfather in the rocking chair next to him, not saying anything, just being there.

The first time he pictured it, it was vague. He breathed. He kept picturing. It got clearer. He could hear the creek. He could smell the pine. He could feel the afternoon sun on his face. His grandfather's calm presence filling the air.

He stayed there for about fifteen minutes, eyes closed, breathing slowly. The plane kept bumping. His body did not stop reacting. But his body was also, for the first time in his adult life, in two places at once. Physically in seat 14A. Mentally on the porch. The porch was winning.

By the time he opened his eyes, the turbulence had eased. He was not calm. But he was not in a panic either. He was a person who had been on a porch for fifteen minutes and had come back to a plane that was now mostly smooth.

What You'll Get From This Chapter

This chapter teaches you the second foundational practice of CFT: safe place imagery. You will learn why imagination is one of the most powerful tools your nervous system has, how to build a safe place that works for your specific body, how to use all five senses to make the image real enough to actually soothe, and what to do when your safe place does not feel safe or when no image comes at all. By the end, you will have a private refuge you can access almost anywhere.

12.1 Why Imagination Works On The Body

Your body does not fully distinguish between what you see in front of you and what you vividly imagine. This is one of the strangest and most useful facts about the human nervous system. When you imagine a lemon, vividly enough, you will often salivate. When you imagine a loved one smiling at you, your body produces some of the same oxytocin it would produce in their actual presence. When you imagine a safe, peaceful place, your body begins to shift toward a settled state, even if you are not in that place (Kreibig, 2010; Holmes & Mathews, 2010).

This is not a loophole. It is a feature. Imagination evolved partly to help us prepare for situations we had not yet encountered, and the preparation included mobilizing the right physical state. Your ancestors who could vividly imagine danger were better prepared for it. Your ancestors who could vividly imagine safety could settle their bodies even in difficult environments. You inherited both capacities.

Modern life uses this system mostly in the wrong direction. You imagine your way into stress regularly. You rehearse an upcoming conversation and your heart speeds up. You remember an embarrassing moment from ten years ago and your face flushes. Your body responds to the imagined scene as if it were happening.

The safe place practice uses the same mechanism, deliberately, in the opposite direction. You build a scene your body reads as safe, and you let your body respond to it. The practice is not escapism. It is using a real physiological tool on purpose.

12.2 Building Your Scene

Your safe place can be anywhere. It can be a real place you have been, a place you have imagined, a composite, or something entirely made up. What matters is that, in the scene, your body reads safety.

Some common starting points: A room from your childhood, if childhood rooms felt safe, A natural setting you have visited (a beach, a meadow, a forest, a lake), A place you have seen only in pictures that appeals to you, A completely imagined place (a garden, a cabin, a cloud, a mountain cave), and A fictional place from a book or film you love, if that feels right.

The place should feel quiet, safe, and nurturing. It should not contain people from your life, at least at first, because people come with complications. You can add a figure later, in Chapter 13.0. For now, just the place.

If you cannot think of one, try this. Close your eyes, breathe slowly for a minute, and let an image come on its own. Do not force it. Many readers find that an image arrives when they stop searching for one. If still nothing comes, try starting with a single element: a sound, a smell, a texture. Build outward from there.

The image does not need to be photo-realistic. It can be vague. It can change each time you visit. It can be cartoonish. It can be mostly a feeling with some fuzzy visual edges. None of this matters. What matters is that your body responds to it as safe.

12.3 Using All Five Senses

The more senses you engage, the more real the scene becomes to your body. Visual imagery alone is less effective than multi-sensory imagery. When you build your safe place, include:

Sight. What do you see? Colors. Light. Shapes. The way the scene is framed. Near things and far things. Time of day.

Sound. What do you hear? Wind. Water. Leaves. Birds. A distant voice. The quiet itself has a sound.

Smell. What do you smell? Pine. Salt air. Bread baking. Rain on dry earth. Coffee. A specific scent from a place you have loved.

Touch. What do you feel on your skin? Sun. Breeze. The texture of a chair. The softness of a blanket. The ground beneath your feet.

Taste. Sometimes this one is harder to include, but if it fits, use it. The taste of tea. The saltiness of sea air. A specific food associated with the place.

You do not need all five every time. Three or four is often enough. The goal is not to build a perfect scene. It is to build a scene that your body recognizes as real enough to respond to.

12.4 A Real Example

Yuki built her safe place slowly. She started with the kitchen of her grandmother's house in Japan, where she had spent summers as a child. For the first few weeks, the image was vague. She could see the wooden table. She could smell the miso soup on the stove. That was about it.

Her therapist encouraged her to add one sense a week. Week two, she added the sound. The kettle whistling. Her grandmother's slippers on the floor. The clock ticking. Week three, she added the light. Late afternoon, golden, coming through a paper screen. Week four, the touch. The warmth of the tea cup in her hands. The texture of the cushion on her chair.

By the end of six weeks, the scene was vivid. She could spend ten minutes there with her eyes closed and feel as if she had actually visited. When she returned to the room, her body was settled. Her shoulders were down. Her breathing was slow.

Her therapist asked her, once the image was strong, to notice something. When Yuki was in her grandmother's kitchen, her critic was quiet. The voice that had been running her life for thirty years went silent. Not because she had fought it. Because the image produced a physiological state the critic could not operate in. The critic lives in threat. The kitchen was green.

This is one of the most useful by-products of the safe place practice. The critic gets quiet because the nervous system it runs on has shifted.

Yuki started using the practice in specific situations. Before difficult meetings. After hard conversations. On Sunday evenings when her anxiety about the coming week would start to rise. Over the course of a year, the practice became automatic. She could drop into her grandmother's kitchen in about ninety seconds.

What this means for you: A safe place built slowly, with multi-sensory detail, becomes more than a nice image. It becomes a reliable physiological tool. The richer the detail, the stronger the effect. You are not just visualizing. You are giving your body a full package of safety signals it can respond to.

12.5 Another Real Example

David is forty-four, a veteran. He has complex PTSD. When his first therapist asked him to imagine a safe place, his body rejected every attempt. He tried a beach. The beach felt exposed. He tried a forest. The forest felt like someone could hide in it. He tried his own childhood bedroom. Memories came up that he had spent thirty years not thinking about.

His therapist, who was trauma-informed, changed the approach. She did not ask David to build a safe place. She asked him to find a safer place than the one he was currently in. Just a small step. Not peace. Not comfort. Just somewhat safer.

David tried again. He pictured the cab of his pickup truck, parked in the driveway of his own house, with the engine off. Nothing around him. Windows up. Quiet. He could see the dashboard. He could feel the seat. He was alone. He was contained. He was, marginally, safer than in a public setting.

That was the start. For six months, his safe place was his truck. He did not try to make it a meadow. He did not try to make it beautiful. It was a truck. It worked.

Slowly, over the next year, the truck expanded. He added a fishing spot he had been to once in Montana, reached from the truck. Eventually, he could spend time in the meadow near the water. Eventually, he could imagine a small cabin. The progression took time. Each expansion happened when the previous one had become fully safe.

Now, five years later, David has a safe place that includes the cabin, the meadow, the water, and his dog lying beside him. It did not start there. It started in a truck. And that was enough.

What this means for you: If the conventional safe place (beach, meadow, forest) does not work for your body, do not force it. Start with whatever your body actually reads as safer than where you are. It may be small. It may be odd. It may not look like the safe places in self-help books. That is fine. Your body knows what safe means for you. Follow its lead.

12.6 Full Practice Instructions

Here is the full practice. Read it through once, then try it.

1. Sit upright in a chair, feet on the floor, hands resting on your thighs. Soften your face. Close your eyes or lower your gaze.

2. Begin five minutes of soothing rhythm breathing. Do not rush this. The practice does not land without the breath.

3. Once your body has settled slightly, begin to bring your safe place to mind. Do not force the image. Let it arrive.

4. Start with whichever sense comes easiest. If you see the place first, begin with sight. If you hear it first, begin with sound. Work outward from the first sense to the others.

5. Spend time with each sense. What do you see in detail? What do you hear? What do you smell? What do you feel on your skin? What, if anything, do you taste? Let the scene fill in.

6. Notice how your body is responding. Is there a softening in your chest? A loosening in your shoulders? A slowing of your breath? Let the responses happen. Do not try to make more happen than is happening.

7. Stay in the place for as long as you want. Five minutes. Ten. Twenty, if the session is long. There is no right length.

8. When you are ready to leave, bring your attention back to the room. Notice three things you can hear in your actual environment. Open your eyes. Notice three things you can see.

The return matters. You want to leave the safe place deliberately, not stumble out of it. A clean return makes the practice feel like a completed arc rather than an interrupted one.

12.7 When It Doesn't Work

Several things can go wrong with the safe place practice. Here are the common ones and what to do.

The image keeps shifting. This is very normal, especially early on. A beach becomes a forest becomes a room. Let it shift. You are not failing. The nervous system is exploring what feels safe. Over time, one image usually stabilizes.

The image unsettles you. Memories come up. Old feelings arrive. The place does not feel safe at all. This often means the image is linked to something your body has not fully processed. Gently let that image go. Try a completely different kind of place, or try the David approach (something safer than now, not ideal safe).

You cannot picture anything. Some people have limited visual imagination. This is called aphantasia when it is extreme, and it does not mean you cannot do the practice. Focus on the other senses. Feel the place. Hear it. Smell it. You do not need to see it clearly to be there.

The critic shows up. It says, "You are making this up. This is silly. This is not real." Notice. Name it. Return to the practice. The critic hates safe places because safe places threaten its job.

You feel guilty for being somewhere pleasant while the world is hard. Some readers, especially those with high baseline responsibility, feel undeserving of peace. This is a sign of how under-nourished your soothing system has been. You do not have to earn your safe place. You can simply go there.

If the practice repeatedly triggers intense distress, please work with a trauma-informed therapist. Some nervous systems need human company to build safety for the first time. There is no failure in this. The practice will still be available once the foundation is laid.

12.8 What To Take Away

Your imagination is a real tool. Your body responds to what you vividly imagine as if it were partially real. This is the foundation of the safe place practice.

Your safe place can be anywhere. Real, imagined, composite, vague. What matters is that your body reads it as safe. Include as many senses as you can, one at a time, building slowly.

The practice starts with soothing rhythm breathing. Always. Without the breath, the imagery has nowhere to land. With the breath, the imagery becomes a reliable tool your body can use.

If the conventional safe places do not work, start smaller. Find something that is safer than now. Build outward from there. There is no right scene. Your body knows what works. Follow it.

For this week, build your safe place slowly. Start with one sense. Add another. By the end of the week, you should have a place you can visit in about three minutes. Visit it once a day. Notice what happens to your body when you are there.

In the next chapter, you will add a figure to your safe place. Or not. You will learn how to create a compassionate other, which is the third major practice in CFT. That practice builds directly on the safe place. Keep going.

Chapter 13: Imagining A Compassionate Other

Michael had been doing the safe place practice for six weeks. It was working. His grandmother's garden, the one from the house he had not visited in thirty years. He could be there in two minutes. His body settled. The critic got quiet. The practice had become reliable.

His therapist introduced the next step in their seventh session. She asked him to imagine, inside the garden, a being who was deeply compassionate. Someone or something that embodied wisdom, strength, warmth, and caring commitment. Someone who was completely and unconditionally for him.

Michael closed his eyes. He tried.

The first person who came to mind was his grandmother herself. He felt a flicker of warmth. Then, almost immediately, he remembered the last conversation they had had before she died, when she had been irritable with him about something small. The warmth collapsed.

He tried his mother. A wave of complicated grief came up. He pushed past it and tried his college roommate. He tried a teacher from high school. He tried a kind neighbor. Each person he brought into the garden came with history, and history came with limits, and limits meant they were not unconditionally for him.

He opened his eyes, frustrated. "I cannot do this one. Every person I think of has some problem."

His therapist smiled gently. "It does not have to be a person."

Michael blinked. He had assumed, without thinking about it, that the compassionate other had to be human. A real figure from his life or one he could imagine as a person. He had never considered any other possibility.

His therapist continued. "It can be an animal. A being of light. A presence without a form. A tree. An ocean. A star. A mythical figure. Anything your body reads as unconditionally compassionate. Because you are inventing this, you can make it whatever will work."

Michael closed his eyes again. He was quiet for a long time. Then something came. A great stag, standing in the garden, with enormous dark eyes and a stillness that felt ancient. It had not moved. It was just there, looking at him, in a way that felt older than words. It was not from his life. It was not anyone he had ever met. It was entirely made up. And his body recognized it instantly as safe.

What You'll Get From This Chapter

This chapter teaches you the third major CFT practice: the compassionate other, sometimes called the ideal compassionate image or the perfect nurturer. You will learn why this practice is so powerful, how to create a figure that works for your specific nervous system, what qualities your compassionate other needs to have, and what to do when real people from your past keep showing up in the image. By the end, you will have a figure you can turn to when your own self-compassion is not yet strong enough.

13.1 Why We Need This Practice

Compassion, in humans, develops largely through receiving it. The soothing system is built in early childhood through contact with caregivers who offer consistent warmth. If you received that, your system has an internal model of being cared for, and you can draw on it later to offer care to yourself. If you did not receive that, or received it inconsistently, your system has little to go on (Mikulincer & Shaver, 2007; Lee, 2005).

The compassionate other practice solves this problem, partially, by giving you a figure you can receive compassion from, regardless of what you did or did not receive in your actual life. Your imagination builds a source of care that your nervous system can respond to. Over time, this imagined source becomes an internal resource you can call on when you need it.

This is not a replacement for human connection. It is a supplement. The compassionate other gives your system a felt sense of being cared for that can exist alongside, and often before, real human care becomes available. Many readers find that after practicing with an imagined compassionate other for several months, they become more able to receive compassion from actual humans in their lives, because the pathway for receiving has been opened.

The practice also gives you a stable figure in a way real people cannot. Real people have bad days. Real people get busy. Real people die, move away, get sick, or become distant. Your compassionate other is always available. This is not a flaw of the practice. It is one of its central gifts.

13.2 The Qualities Your Figure Needs

For the compassionate other practice to work, your figure needs four qualities. These are the same four qualities you met in the compassionate self chapter, now embodied in an external figure. Spending time building each quality deliberately makes the figure more real and more effective (Gilbert, 2009).

Wisdom. Your compassionate other understands how suffering works. They know that life is hard. They know that your struggles are not your fault. They do not blame. They see clearly.

Strength. Your compassionate other does not collapse when things get difficult. They do not flinch at your pain. They can hold the full weight of what you are carrying without being overwhelmed. They are steady.

Warmth. Your compassionate other feels genuine care for you. Not polite interest. Not professional concern. A deep, felt warmth. The kind of warmth you would recognize as real if you encountered it.

Caring commitment. Your compassionate other is fully on your side. They want your wellbeing. They will not abandon you. They will not judge you. They are committed to you, no matter what.

When you build your figure, spend time with each quality. Let the figure embody all four. Feel what it is like to be in the presence of a being who is wise, strong, warm, and committed to you. Your body will recognize it. Your body knows what this feels like, even if you have never experienced it from a real human.

13.3 Building The Figure

Here is how to begin. You will refine the image over time.

Form. What form does your figure take? A person (real or imagined). An animal. A being of light. A tree. A mountain. A wave. An ancestor figure. A god or goddess. A fictional character. A mythological being. Something you have never seen and cannot name. Anything is allowed. Let the form arrive. Do not edit it.

Presence. How does the figure feel? Not what does it look like, but what is the felt sense of being near it? Calm? Vast?

Steady? Old? Warm? Every figure has a presence, and often the presence is more important than the visual.

Eyes. If the figure has eyes, what are they like? Compassionate eyes are a specific thing. They hold you without judgment. They see you without recoiling. They convey, without words, that you are known and accepted.

Voice. If the figure speaks, what is the voice like? Pace. Tone. Warmth. Depth. Some figures do not speak with words; they communicate through presence alone. That is fine.

Relationship to you. What is the figure's relationship to you? Some figures feel like a wise grandparent. Some feel like a protective animal guardian. Some feel like a divine being. Some feel like an older, wiser version of yourself. There is no right relationship.

You do not need to answer all of these at once. Let the figure develop over several sessions. Each time you practice, spend a minute or two letting the figure fill in more.

13.4 A Real Example

Mary, the lawyer from Chapter 8.0, tried the compassionate other practice after her breakdown in the garage. She had been doing the safe place practice for a few weeks. Her safe place was a cabin in the mountains she had visited once on a long weekend.

Her first attempt at a compassionate other did not work. She tried her grandmother. Her grandmother had been kind, but also Catholic and fairly judgmental about Mary's career choices. The image came with history. Mary could not fully let her in.

She tried her college mentor. Same problem. The mentor had retired and Mary had lost touch. The distance felt like a subtle rejection, even though it was not.

Her therapist suggested trying a completely invented figure. Someone who had no history with Mary at all, because they did not exist.

Mary tried. At first, nothing came. Then, slowly, a figure began to take shape. A woman, tall, with long silver hair, standing in the cabin. She wore simple clothes. She was older than Mary, but not frail. Her eyes were calm and kind. She did not smile widely. She conveyed, through her steady presence, that she had seen a lot of life and that nothing Mary could share would shock her or push her away.

Mary named her, though the therapist had not suggested it. She called her Ida. Ida became Mary's compassionate other for the next three years. Ida did not give advice. Ida did not solve problems. Ida sat with Mary, in the cabin, and by her presence alone, communicated that Mary was not alone and that whatever she was carrying was allowed to exist.

What Mary found, over time, was that Ida's voice began to show up in her daily life, without being summoned. At a moment of high stress in a courtroom, she would hear, in her own mind, a phrase Ida might have said. Nothing dramatic. Just a steady, "You are all right. You can slow down." The figure had become an internalized resource, a voice Mary could call on without needing to sit down and do a full practice.

That is the purpose of the practice. Not to depend on the image forever. To internalize the quality of care the image carries, so that eventually, the quality becomes part of you.

What this means for you: Your compassionate other does not have to be based on anyone you have known. In fact, for many readers, a completely invented figure works better than a real one, because invented figures come without history, complication, or disappointment. Let your imagination do the work. Trust what arrives.

13.5 The Full Practice

Here is the full practice. Read through once, then try it.

1. Settle into your chair. Soft face. Upright posture. Hands on thighs.

2. Do five minutes of soothing rhythm breathing. Let your body settle.

3. Bring your safe place to mind. Let the scene fill in with as many senses as you can. Spend two or three minutes fully arriving.

4. Now invite your compassionate other into the scene. If you have a figure already, bring them in. If you do not yet, let one arrive. Do not force the image. Let it come on its own.

5. Notice your figure. What do they look like? What is their presence? What are their eyes like? What is the feeling of being in their company?

6. Let them look at you. Feel their eyes on you. Feel their warmth. Feel their complete acceptance of you, exactly as you are.

7. If they speak, listen. If they are silent, let the silence be full. Presence without words is often more powerful than words.

8. You may want to tell them something. A struggle. A grief. A moment from the day. Speak, silently or aloud. Notice how they receive it. Notice that they do not flinch, do not judge, do not rush to fix.

9. Stay in their presence for as long as you want. Ten minutes. Twenty. The time does not matter. The contact does.

10. When you are ready, thank them silently. Know that they are always available. Let the image fade. Come back to the breath. Open your eyes.

13.6 Another Real Example

Layla, whose childhood had been chaotic and whose soothing system was barely developed, had the hardest time with this practice of any she had tried. For the first month, every figure she imagined felt untrustworthy. She would build a figure, and within seconds, her mind would generate reasons the figure was not safe. The figure might be kind now, but what about later. The figure might care, but what about when it mattered. The figure was in her head, so the figure was just her, so how could the figure be trusted any more than she trusted herself.

She almost gave up.

Her therapist suggested something she had not thought of. The therapist asked Layla to think of a moment in her life, any moment, when she had felt unconditionally welcomed by a living being. Just one moment.

Layla thought for a long time. She finally remembered a stray cat who had adopted her during a bad summer. The cat had shown up at her door one night and stayed for about three months before disappearing. The cat had asked nothing of her. The cat had sat on her lap in the evenings. The cat had slept at the foot of her bed. When Layla had cried, the cat had come over and sat near her.

The therapist asked, "Can the cat be your compassionate other?"

Layla laughed, then cried. Yes. The cat could.

She named the cat Muffin, which was what she had called her at the time. Muffin became her compassionate other. Not a human figure. Not a wise elder. A small gray cat with green eyes, who had actually, in real life, once offered Layla unconditional presence without demanding anything in return.

Muffin worked. Muffin's presence bypassed all of Layla's trust issues with humans, because Muffin was not a human, and because Muffin had, at one time, been real. The figure had a memory of actual safety to draw on.

Over years of practice, Layla's compassionate other slowly expanded. Muffin remained. Other figures joined her. Eventually, an older woman showed up in the image, gentle and unhurried. Layla trusted her because Muffin had trusted her first.

What this means for you: If humans do not work as your compassionate other, animals often do. If neither works, consider a nature element (a tree, the ocean, the stars). If even that is hard, think back to any moment in your life where you felt safely received, by anyone or anything, and let that moment be the seed of your figure. The figure can grow from there.

13.7 When It Doesn't Work

Several things commonly go wrong with this practice. Here are the fixes.

You cannot picture any figure at all. Focus on presence rather than image. What would the feeling of being fully accepted be like? Build from that feeling, not from a visual. The figure may emerge slowly, over weeks.

Every figure you try feels wrong. This often means you are trying to use real people, and every real person comes with history. Try an invented figure. Try an animal. Try a being of light with no form at all.

The figure feels fake. This is very common early on. The practice will feel artificial for the first several weeks. You are essentially acting out a scene with a figure who does not exist. Your rational mind will protest. Keep going. The body responds to the figure even when the mind calls it fake. Over time, the mind catches up.

The figure's voice sounds like your critic. This means the figure has been hijacked by your threat system. The critic does not want you to have an alternative voice. Notice what happened. Start the practice over. Make the figure explicitly gentle, warm, non-judging. If the critic keeps breaking through, the issue is usually not the figure. It is that you are trying to do the practice when your threat system is already too activated. Do more breathing first.

You feel overwhelmed by emotion. Unexpected grief or tears can come up, especially for readers who did not receive unconditional care in childhood. The figure is giving you something you have been missing. Let the emotion move. This is not a problem with the practice. This is the practice working.

If any of this becomes unmanageable, a trauma-informed therapist can hold the practice with you. Some nervous systems need human company to meet this particular figure for the first time. There is no shame in that. The practice is powerful precisely because it points at something real.

13.8 Before You Move On

Your compassionate other is a figure you build in your imagination who embodies wisdom, strength, warmth, and caring commitment. Their job is to be fully on your side, unconditionally, forever.

The figure can take any form. Human, animal, nature, being of light, mythological figure, something entirely invented. What matters is that your body reads them as safe and as caring. Real people from your past often do not work well, because they come with history. Invented figures often work better.

The practice builds on soothing rhythm breathing and the safe place. Breathe first. Arrive in the safe place. Let the figure join you. Receive their presence. This is the sequence. Without the breath and the place, the figure has nothing to anchor to.

Over months of practice, the figure becomes internalized. Their voice begins to show up in your daily life without being called. This is the goal. The practice is a training. The internalization is the graduation.

For this week, spend ten minutes a day building and meeting your compassionate other. If a figure does not arrive in the first few sessions, that is normal. Keep the appointment with yourself. The figure will come.

In the next chapter, you will learn compassionate letter writing. Letters are where the internal figure begins to have a voice on paper, which is different from a voice in the head. Many readers report that this practice, more than any other, changes their relationship with themselves. Keep going.

Chapter 14: Writing Yourself A Kind Letter

Zara sat at her kitchen table at 9 p.m. on a Sunday. A blank notebook was open in front of her. A cup of tea was going cold next to it. She had been staring at the page for about ten minutes.

Her therapist had given her an assignment. Write a letter to yourself from your compassionate other. Any length. Any topic. Just write.

Zara had not written a real letter to anyone in years. Texts, emails, work memos. No letters. Certainly no letters to herself. The exercise felt silly. She almost put the notebook away.

Instead, she tried something. She wrote, at the top of the page: "Dear Zara." Then she stopped. The word "Dear" looked strange. She considered crossing it out. She left it.

She began. "I wanted to write to you about today." She paused. She did not know what else to say.

She kept going. "Today was hard. You got home and went straight to bed for two hours without eating. You did not even take off your shoes. You scrolled on your phone and felt more and more tired. When you finally got up, you were too tired to cook, so you ate cereal standing at the counter."

She noticed something. She had started writing from her own voice, not from the compassionate other. She tried to switch. She imagined the stag figure her therapist had been working with her on. She tried to write as the stag would speak, if the stag spoke.

"The day was hard," she wrote, "and you kept going. You did the meeting. You responded to the email. You handled your mother's phone call. You were exhausted, and you still did those things. You did not fail today. You survived a hard day. Survival is not nothing."

She stopped. She read what she had written. She started to cry, quietly, sitting at her kitchen table with her cold tea.

The words were not profound. She would not have read them back in a book and thought much of them. But she had written them to herself, as someone who saw her and was not judging her, and no one had spoken to her that way in a very long time. Maybe ever. She cried for about ten minutes. Then she wrote three more paragraphs. Then she put the notebook away and went to bed. She slept better than she had in weeks.

What You'll Get From This Chapter

This chapter teaches you the compassionate letter writing practice, which is one of the most evidence-based tools in CFT. You will learn why writing is different from thinking, how to structure a letter that actually lands, what a compassionate voice on paper sounds like, and what to do with the letters after you write them. You will see a full worked example of a letter, with commentary on what makes it compassionate rather than self-pitying or self-critical. By the end, you will have a practice you can return to weekly for the rest of your life.

14.1 Why Writing Is Different From Thinking

Thoughts move fast. They loop. They interrupt each other. They get hijacked by the critic before they finish forming. Writing slows everything down. You can only write one word at a time. The pace alone is therapeutic (Pennebaker, 1997).

Writing also forces specificity. When you think, "I had a hard day," the thought can be vague, abstract, unexamined. When you write, "I had a hard day," your pen wants to know what made it hard. You have to say. The writing extracts detail that thinking leaves buried.

Writing creates a witness. When you write a letter to yourself from a compassionate voice, you are producing an artifact. A piece of paper with kind words on it that exists outside your head. You can come back to it tomorrow. You can read it to yourself when you are struggling. You can see, in your own handwriting, that someone (you) saw the struggle clearly and responded with care.

Writing, especially hand-writing, also engages more of your nervous system than thinking does. The physical act of forming letters, the sensation of pen on paper, the visual of the words appearing, all contribute to a sense of realness. Research has consistently shown that expressive writing produces measurable benefits for mood, stress, and even physical health (Pennebaker & Smyth, 2016). Compassionate letter writing takes that foundation and adds a specific therapeutic aim.

14.2 How To Start

Here is the basic structure of a compassionate letter. It is not a formula. It is a scaffold you can adapt.

Set up the practice. Sit somewhere quiet. Pen and paper, ideally, though typing works if writing is physically hard for you. Spend five minutes in soothing rhythm breathing to settle your body. Briefly bring your compassionate other to mind. You are going to write from their voice.

Begin with a greeting. "Dear [your name]," works fine. Some readers feel that "Dear" is too formal. You can use "Hi," or "Hello," or skip the greeting entirely. What matters is that you are being addressed, by someone, specifically.

Acknowledge what is hard. Not in a dramatic way. In a specific, honest way. What has been difficult lately? What has the person been carrying? Name it plainly. "Today was hard because X." "This week has been heavy." "You have been dealing with Y and it is a lot."

Validate, without minimizing. This is where the compassionate voice differs from the critic. The critic says, "You should be over this by now." The compassionate voice says, "What you are feeling makes sense, given what you are going through." Validation is not agreement with every thought. It is acknowledgment that the feelings have a legitimate source.

Name what the person has done well. Often, in hard times, the accomplishment is simply surviving. "You kept going. You showed up. You did not give up, even when it felt like you might." Small things count. The critic dismisses these. The compassionate voice sees them.

Offer perspective. Gently, without lecturing. "This is one moment in a longer life. The hard feelings will shift. You have moved through hard things before." Perspective is not a demand to feel better. It is a reminder that the current state is not the whole picture.

Close with presence. Not a solution. Just presence. "I am here. I see you. I am not going anywhere." A short closing line that signals the compassionate voice will remain available.

Sign off. "With love," "With care," or some version that feels right. Sign it with a name. It can be your own name (the compassionate part of you signing to the struggling part). It can be the name of your compassionate other. It can be something symbolic.

The whole letter takes fifteen to thirty minutes. It does not have to be long. A one-page letter is plenty.

14.3 A Real Example Letter

Here is a full letter written by Isabella, the physician from Chapter 6.0, during a particularly hard stretch. She shared it with her therapist, who shared it (with her permission) as an example. Names have been changed.

Dear Isabella,

I am writing to you tonight because I know it has been a brutal week. The Monday case hit hard, harder than the ones before it, and I know you are still carrying it. You did not sleep Tuesday. You cried in the supply closet Wednesday before clinic. You have been snappish with Jorge and with the kids. You have not been kind to yourself about any of it.

I want to say some things that I do not think you have let yourself hear.

First: what happened Monday was not your fault. You know this, somewhere, but your mind has been running the case a hundred times looking for the moment you should have caught something. Medicine does not work that way. You did what any of your colleagues would have done, and what you did was good care. The outcome was not something you controlled. This is the hardest part of your job, and it has always been the hardest part.

Second: you are allowed to grieve. You have been treating this week as a weakness to get through. It is not a weakness. It is grief, for a patient, in a job that asks you to give real care and then tells you to move on when the care does not work. Of course you are tired. Of course you are tender. Of course you are not sleeping.

Third: you have been doing this for ten years, and you have helped more people than you can count. Hundreds of families have been better off because of you. That is not erased by one case. That is not a ledger that resets. You have a long history of doing this work with skill and with heart. This week does not undo any of that.

I am not telling you to snap out of it. I am telling you that what you are feeling makes sense, and that you are not failing for feeling it. I am also telling you that you have earned rest. You are allowed to go to bed early. You are allowed to skip the gym. You are allowed to tell Jorge that you need a quiet evening. None of that will set you back.

The week will pass. This feeling will shift. You have moved through hard weeks before, and you will move through this one. The only thing I want from you right now is that you eat something before bed, and that you let yourself cry if you need to cry. Both are allowed.

I am here. I see all of this. I am not going anywhere.

With love, Isabella

Notice a few things about this letter. It is specific. It names the actual situation. It validates the feelings without minimizing them. It offers some perspective without demanding that Isabella feel different. It makes room for grief. It ends with presence, not a prescription. It is signed by her own name, because Isabella decided that her compassionate voice was part of her, not a separate being.

Your letter does not have to look like this one. It can be shorter. It can be less polished. It can be messier. What matters is the voice and the witnessing.

14.4 The Compassionate Voice

Learning to hear the compassionate voice in your own head, in real time, is the long project of this work. For the letter, you can start more simply. Ask yourself: how would I speak to a good friend who was going through exactly what I am going through?

That is the voice. That is what the letter uses. Not the voice you use with yourself by default. The voice you already have, which you use for other people, which you can borrow for one page.

Some readers find it helps to imagine the letter is being written to a close friend with the same situation, and then, once it is written, to change the name at the top to their own. The voice comes easier when the reader is someone else. The trick works.

Things to include in the voice: Specific acknowledgment of what is hard, Phrases like "it makes sense that..." or "given what you are carrying...", Recognition of what the person has done or endured, Gentle perspective, not lecturing, Permission to feel what they are feeling, and Presence, not fixing.

Things to avoid: "You should..." or "You need to..." (lecturing), "At least..." (minimizing), "Other people have it worse..." (comparison), "You brought this on yourself..." (blaming), "If you had just..." (criticizing), and "Everything happens for a reason..." (dismissing).

When the critic tries to hijack the letter, you will notice. The tone will shift. The words will get harder. Cross out that paragraph and start again. You do not have to be perfect. You just have to notice when the voice changes and steer it back.

14.5 Another Real Example

Omar started the letter writing practice with deep skepticism. He was an engineer. Writing felt foreign. The idea of writing to himself felt especially foreign. He did it because his therapist had asked him to.

His first letter was four sentences long. He read it back and hated it. It sounded stiff. It sounded like a performance. He almost threw it away. He did not. He put it in a folder.

His second letter, a week later, was a little longer. Still stiff. Still felt fake. He kept going. His third letter was seven sentences, and in it, he wrote one line that surprised him. He wrote, "I know you are tired, and I know nobody has said that out loud to you in a long time."

He stared at that line for a while. He put the notebook away.

Over the next six months, he wrote a letter every Sunday night. The letters got longer. The voice got warmer. By month four, the letters had become something he looked forward to. By month six, he was writing to himself in difficult moments during the week, not just on Sundays. He would pull out his notebook and write half a page in his car before walking into a meeting he was dreading.

Here is the change he reported. "I used to talk to myself like a drill sergeant. Now I talk to myself like a coach who actually wants me to win. The coach is still tough when I need it. But the coach is on my side. That is new."

Omar kept all his letters. At the end of the year, he read the first one again. The stiff, four-sentence one he had almost thrown away. He realized, reading it, that even that first awkward attempt had a kindness in it he had not been able to see at the time. The first letter was the seed. The ones that came after were the growth.

What this means for you: Your first letters will probably be awkward. They will feel fake. Keep them anyway. The practice is about the repetition, not about the quality of any single letter. The voice grows over months, not over one night.

14.6 How Often And What To Do After

For most readers, once a week is the right rhythm. A full letter, fifteen to thirty minutes, typically on the same day and time each week. Sunday evenings, before bed, work well for many. Find a rhythm that fits your life.

Shorter letters can be written more often. Three or four sentences in a notebook, during a difficult moment. These do not replace the weekly full letter, but they can supplement it.

Keep your letters. Do not throw them away. A physical notebook is ideal. A dedicated note on your phone is fine. The letters are a record of your own compassionate voice growing over time. When you read them back after a year, you will see patterns. You will see how your voice has evolved. You will see struggles that felt huge at the time and have since softened. The letters become their own form of evidence that you are changing.

Some readers read old letters when they are struggling. This can be powerful. A letter you wrote to yourself eight months ago, addressing exactly what you are struggling with now, can land harder than any book or podcast, because it was written by someone (you) who knew you.

You can also, occasionally, read a letter out loud to yourself. Hearing the compassionate voice in your own literal voice is a strange and powerful experience. Some readers find it awkward at first. Most find that it deepens the practice significantly.

14.7 When It Doesn't Work

Several things can go wrong with the letter practice. Common ones:

The letter sounds fake. This is universal at first. The voice is new. Writing in a voice you have not used before will feel performed. Keep writing. The voice settles into itself over weeks.

The critic writes the letter. Halfway through a letter, you notice the tone has shifted. The letter is now lecturing you, blaming you, telling you to try harder. This is the critic grabbing the pen. Stop. Notice. Cross out the paragraph. Start over with your compassionate voice. You do not have to be perfect. You just have to notice the takeover and steer back.

You do not know what to write. Many readers freeze in front of the blank page. Here is a trick. Start with the phrase: "I want to write to you about..." Then finish the sentence honestly. Whatever is heavy. Whatever is on your mind. The beginning does not have to be elegant. The letter unfolds once you start.

You feel silly. You are writing to yourself, and some part of you is rolling its eyes. That is fine. You can write while feeling silly. The nervous system does not care if you feel silly. The practice still works.

You cry when you write. This is common, especially for readers who did not receive compassion in childhood. The letter gives you something you have been missing. Grief is one of the natural responses. Let it come. The crying is part of the healing, not a disruption to it.

You avoid writing. You know the practice is useful. You do not write. Weeks go by. The resistance is itself a form of data. It usually means the practice is pointing at something tender. Lower the bar. Write three sentences. Not a full letter. Three sentences are enough. Start there.

If the letter practice consistently produces intense distress that you cannot move through, please work with a therapist. Some letters uncover material that needs more support than a page can provide.

14.8 Pulling It Together

Compassionate letter writing is one of the most powerful practices in CFT. It slows down the compassionate voice. It creates an artifact of your kindness toward yourself that exists outside your head. It produces a record, over months and years, of your own growth.

The structure is simple. Greet yourself. Acknowledge what is hard. Validate without minimizing. Name what you have done or endured. Offer gentle perspective. Close with presence. Sign. Fifteen to thirty minutes. Once a week is a good rhythm.

The voice is the voice you would use with a friend. Not the voice you default to with yourself. You already have it. The practice is about redirecting it.

Your first letters will feel fake. Keep them anyway. The voice grows over months. By the end of a year of weekly letters, you will have something rare: a body of evidence, in your own handwriting, that you are capable of being kind to yourself. That evidence is one of the things that, over time, quiets the critic.

For this week, write one letter. Fifteen minutes. Any topic. Any length. Put it in a folder. Next week, write another. Do not evaluate the letters. Do not grade them. Just write them. The cumulative effect is the point.

In the next chapter, you will learn to work with your inner critic directly, using everything you have built so far. The critic will still show up. But now, you will have tools.

Chapter 15: Working With The Inner Critic

Maria had been arguing with her critic for most of her life. She knew the arguments by heart. The critic would say something cutting. Maria would counter. The critic would counter the counter. Twenty minutes later, Maria would be exhausted, the critic would have won, and Maria would have nothing to show for it except a worse mood than when she started.

Tonight was different. It was 10 p.m. on a Thursday. Her critic was going at her about a conversation she had had with her sister that afternoon. The conversation had been fine. The critic was not letting it be fine. *You were too defensive. You sounded petty. She probably thinks you are ridiculous. You always do this. You always come across as insecure.*

Maria caught herself about to start the old argument. *I was not petty. We were just talking about Mom.* She stopped. She had read a chapter the week before that had suggested a different approach. She decided to try it.

She sat down at her desk. She got a piece of paper. She wrote, at the top: "What my critic just said." Then she wrote, in full sentences, what the critic had been saying. She did not edit. She did not soften. She wrote it all out.

Looking at it on paper, she noticed something. The critic was not making a case. The critic was attacking. The critic was saying things that, if anyone else had said them to her, Maria would have gotten up and walked out of the room. The critic had been saying those things to her for decades, and she had been staying.

She took another sheet of paper. She wrote, at the top: "What my critic is actually scared of." She thought for a while. She wrote:

"The critic is scared that my sister does not love me. The critic is scared I will end up alone. The critic thinks if it points out everything I did wrong, I will do it better next time, and then I will not be rejected."

She looked at that page for a long time. The critic was not her enemy. The critic was a scared child who had learned, somewhere, that attack was the only way to keep Maria safe. The critic had been doing it for so long that it did not know how to stop.

She took a third sheet. She wrote, at the top: "What my compassionate self would say to this critic." She began to write. She did not write to herself. She wrote to the critic. She said: "You have been working really hard. You are exhausted. You have been trying to keep me safe in a way that has not worked for a long time. You do not have to work this hard anymore."

She cried a little. She put the three pages away. She went to bed. The critic was still there. But Maria was no longer fighting it, and she was no longer obeying it. Something else had become possible.

What You'll Get From This Chapter

This chapter pulls together everything you have built in Part Four. You will learn how to work with your inner critic, using soothing rhythm breathing, the compassionate self, and letter writing as the foundation. You will see why arguing with the critic does not work, why finding the critic's fear changes everything, and how to have a dialogue with the critic that neither fights it nor obeys it. By the end, you will have a method you can use whenever the critic shows up, which will be often, for the rest of your life.

15.1 Why Arguing Does Not Work

The most common approach to the inner critic is to argue with it. The critic says you are stupid. You counter that you are not stupid, you have evidence, here are your accomplishments. The critic updates its argument. You update yours. The exchange goes on until one of you gives up, and it is almost never the critic.

This approach fails for a structural reason. The critic is a threat-system strategy. Threat-system strategies do not respond to logic. They respond to safety signals. When you argue with the critic, you are using logic to treat a system that does not speak logic. The critic can keep generating new attacks faster than you can rebut them, because generation is cheap and rebuttal is expensive.

Arguing also has a subtle effect. It reinforces the critic's place as a legitimate voice to engage with. By treating the critic as a debate partner, you are, unintentionally, granting it authority. The critic is not a colleague. The critic is a scared part of you trying to protect you with the only tool it has. You would not debate a scared child. You would help them.

This does not mean you accept what the critic says. It means you stop treating the critic as a voice to defeat and start treating it as a voice to understand. The difference changes everything.

15.2 Finding The Critic's Fear

Underneath every critic attack, there is a fear. The fear is the critic's actual motivation. The attack is just its strategy. If you can find the fear, you can change the conversation (Gilbert, 2010; Whelton & Greenberg, 2005).

Here are some common critic attacks and the fears underneath them:

Attack	Fear Underneath
"You are stupid."	"You will be rejected for seeming incompetent."
"You are lazy."	"You will fail and be exposed as unworthy"
"You are ugly."	"You will not be loved."
"You are selfish."	"You will be rejected for not giving enoug"
"You are too much."	"You will be abandoned for being intense."
"You are not enough."	"You will lose your place in the group."
"You are a failure."	"You will not survive."

Notice that each fear is, at its root, about safety. Connection. Survival. Belonging. These are old, old concerns. The critic is not wrong that these things matter. The critic is just using strategies (attack, shame, contempt) that do not actually produce them.

When you find the critic's fear, something shifts. The critic stops being an attacker and starts being a protector who is terrified. You can still disagree with its methods. You can still choose not to act on its suggestions. But the relationship changes. Compassion becomes possible, because you can see the suffering underneath the attack.

This is not the same as excusing what the critic does. It is also not the same as letting the critic run the show. It is the middle path: seeing the critic clearly, understanding what it is trying to do, and choosing a different response.

15.3 A Real Example

Jennifer (from Chapter 8.0) worked with her critic for months before she found the fear. Her critic was primarily the perfectionist kind. Every piece of work could have been better. Every presentation had a mistake. Every meeting was a partial failure.

Her therapist asked her one session: "If the critic got what it wanted, what would the world look like?"

Jennifer thought for a while. She said, "I would be flawless at everything. I would never make a mistake. I would always be prepared."

The therapist said, "And if you were flawless, what would happen?"

Jennifer opened her mouth to answer. She realized she did not have a good one. She tried anyway. "I would succeed at work."

The therapist pushed gently. "And if you succeeded at work, what would happen?"

"I would be respected."

"And if you were respected, what would happen?"

"I would not be dismissed."

Jennifer stopped. The word "dismissed" had come out of her mouth without planning. She sat with it for a minute. The therapist waited.

Jennifer finally said, "My father dismissed my mother. Her whole life. I watched her try and try, and he still dismissed her. I have been trying to be so good at everything that nobody could ever dismiss me the way he dismissed her."

Her critic was not trying to make her fail. Her critic was trying to make her un-dismissable. The perfectionism was a shield. It had been running since she was about nine, and she had never noticed what it was actually protecting her from.

Once she saw the fear, she could talk to the critic differently. She wrote a letter to her critic. She said, in part: "You have been working hard for a long time to make sure I never become my mother. I see that. I am grateful that you were trying to protect me. The problem is that the strategy has not been working. I have been driving myself into the ground, and I am still scared of being dismissed. Maybe there is a different way."

The critic did not immediately retire. But it got quieter. And Jennifer got clearer about where the voice was coming from, which changed how much weight she gave it.

What this means for you: Your critic is not random. It has a specific fear, and that fear has a specific history. You may not know the history yet. That is fine. You can still find the fear, and finding the fear is more than half the work.

15.4 The Chair Dialogue

One of the most powerful tools for working with the critic is a practice called chair work, adapted here for solo practice at home. The idea is simple: instead of arguing with the critic in your head, you give the critic a chair, and you give your compassionate self a chair, and you let them talk (Gilbert & Irons, 2005; Kellogg, 2015).

Here is the practice:

1. Find two chairs, facing each other. Or one chair and a cushion. You will move between them.

2. Sit in the first chair. This is your critic chair. Let the critic speak. Out loud, if you can. Let it say the full attack. Do not edit. Do not soften. Let the critic say what it says.

3. Get up. Move to the other chair. This is your compassionate self chair. Take a minute to settle. Breathe slowly. Embody the compassionate posture. Let your face soften.

4. From the compassionate self, speak back. Not arguing. Not denying. Listening and responding. You might say: "I hear you. I know you are scared. What are you actually afraid will happen?"

5. Get up. Move back to the critic chair. Let the critic answer the question. This is where the fear often surfaces. The critic, asked what it is afraid of, usually drops the attack tone and says something more vulnerable.

6. Move back to the compassionate self chair. Respond to what the critic just said. Acknowledge its fear. Acknowledge how hard it has been working. Offer a different perspective.

7. Continue the dialogue as long as is useful. Sometimes it is three rounds. Sometimes it is ten. End when something shifts, or when you have reached a natural stopping point.

This practice sounds strange. Doing it feels strange. Many readers find it surprisingly powerful once they try it. The physical act of moving between chairs makes the internal dialogue external and concrete. You can actually hear your own critic's fear in your own voice. You can actually practice your compassionate response, out loud, which is different from imagining it silently.

15.5 Another Real Example

Javier, the pediatrician from Chapter 9.0, did chair work during a particularly hard stretch after his son's diagnosis. His critic was relentless. He was a bad father for not having caught it sooner. He was a bad doctor for not recognizing the signs. He was failing his family.

He did the dialogue. His critic said the attacks. He moved to the compassionate self chair. From there, he asked his critic what it was afraid of.

The critic answered, in his own voice, something that surprised him: "I am afraid that if I am not hard on you, something worse will happen to him. I am afraid that my attack is the only thing keeping me alert. If I stop, he will get worse."

Javier had not expected that answer. He moved back to the compassionate self. He said to his critic: "I understand. You think the attack is what is keeping him alive. You think if you let up, you will miss something. But you are not actually making me more alert. You are making me exhausted. An exhausted father is not a more alert father. He is a less alert one. The attack is not working. What might help would be rest, connection, and real information from the specialists. Those are what will keep him safe. Not your attack."

He sat with that for a while. The critic, he reported, did not disappear. But it got quieter. He was able to sleep that night, for the first time in weeks. And when the critic showed up again the next morning, he recognized it faster and could return to the compassionate voice with less effort.

What this means for you: Chair work surfaces conversations you have been having in the back of your mind for years, and brings them into the light. The answers that come, when the critic is actually asked, are often not what you expect. They are usually softer, more frightened, and more workable than the attacks that were on the surface.

15.6 Not Fighting, Not Obeying

The trap most people fall into with their critic is either fighting it or obeying it. Fighting it leads to exhaustion. Obeying it leads to damage. The middle path is to listen to it, understand it, thank it for its efforts, and then choose your own response.

This sounds simple. It is extremely hard in practice. The critic has decades of momentum. Choosing, in the moment, to neither fight nor obey requires catching the critic at the front end of its attack, which takes practice.

Here is a simple framework you can use when the critic shows up. It has three steps, and you can run it in under a minute.

Step 1: Notice. "The critic is speaking." Just name it. Do not engage yet. Recognize that the voice you are hearing is the critic, not the truth.

Step 2: Ask. "What is the critic afraid of right now?" Pause. Let the fear surface. It may take a few tries. The answer often surprises you.

Step 3: Respond from the compassionate self. "I hear you. I see you are worried about X. Thank you for trying to protect me. I am going to do something different now."

That is the whole move. It takes practice. You will not get it right every time. When you miss, which you will, notice the miss and try again next time. Over months, the three-step response becomes more automatic, and your default relationship with the critic shifts.

15.7 When It Doesn't Work

Several things commonly go wrong when people work with their critics. Here are the fixes.

The critic refuses to say its fear. It keeps attacking. It will not answer the question about what it is afraid of. This usually means your threat system is too activated to let the critic drop its guard. Try doing five minutes of soothing rhythm breathing first, then approach the critic again. The critic is less defensive when the body is settled.

The critic says its fear is true. For example, you ask what it is afraid of, and it says, "I am afraid you actually are a failure." In that case, you are still in the attack layer, not the fear layer. Ask again: "And if I were a failure, what would happen?" Keep asking. The real fear is usually two or three layers below the surface.

The compassionate self sounds fake in the dialogue. Normal at first. Keep doing it. The voice settles.

The chair work feels silly. Many readers feel this. It still works. You can do it without the physical chairs; you can do it in your head. But the physical version is more powerful, because the body is involved. Try it at least once in full, even if you feel silly. Silly and effective are not mutually exclusive.

You find something painful from your past. Chair work can surface old material. If something significant comes up (a memory, an insight into a family pattern, a grief you had not felt before), please take care of yourself. Put the work down. Move gently through the rest of the day. If the material is too big for solo practice, a therapist can help you process it safely.

15.8 The Main Ideas

Arguing with your critic does not work. Your critic does not respond to logic. It responds to understanding. The way to change your relationship with the critic is not to defeat it. It is to hear what it is afraid of, and to respond from a different voice.

Every critic has a fear underneath its attack. The attack is the strategy. The fear is the actual concern, and the fear is almost always about safety, belonging, or survival. Finding the fear changes the relationship. You stop seeing the critic as an enemy and start seeing it as a scared part of you using old strategies.

The chair dialogue is one of the most powerful tools for this work. Two chairs, a dialogue between the critic and the compassionate self, out loud or internally. The physical movement between chairs makes the internal external, which makes change possible.

The three-step in-the-moment framework is: notice, ask, respond. Notice when the critic speaks. Ask what it is afraid of. Respond from the compassionate self. You will miss many times. Keep practicing.

For this week, try one chair dialogue. Set aside twenty minutes. Two chairs. Actual movement. Let the critic speak. Ask it what it is afraid of. Respond from your compassionate self. Notice what comes up. Write about it afterward if you want.

This chapter closes Part Four. You have now learned the five foundational practices of CFT: soothing rhythm breathing, safe place imagery, the compassionate other, compassionate letter writing, and working with the inner critic. Any one of these can take months to fully develop. Together, over time, they rewire how you relate to your own suffering.

Part Five comes next. It addresses what happens when the practices do not work, when being kind to yourself makes you feel worse, or when your past gets in the way. These are real challenges, and the next two chapters address them honestly. Keep going. You are further than you were when you started.

PART V: WHEN IT GETS HARD

172

Chapter 16: Backdraft And Why It Hurts

Anya had been doing the practices for three weeks. She had been skeptical at the start, and the first two weeks had confirmed her skepticism. Nothing had happened. She had sat in her chair. She had breathed. She had imagined the compassionate other (a large willow tree in a meadow). She had felt, mostly, a mild sense of boredom.

On the Tuesday of week three, something different happened. She was doing the practice. The willow was steady. Her breath was slow. A simple phrase drifted into her mind, the way phrases sometimes do during practice. "You have been working so hard."

The phrase hit her like a truck.

She started sobbing. Not gentle crying. The kind of crying that bends a person over at the waist. She was heaving for breath. She was making sounds she had not made since she was a child. She stayed like that for maybe eight minutes, on the floor of her living room, with the dog watching her from the corner, alarmed.

When it finally passed, she was shaking. She felt wrung out. She was also furious. What had happened to her? She had been sitting in a chair, imagining a tree, saying a kind sentence to herself. That was not supposed to produce a meltdown. That was supposed to produce calm. She had clearly broken something.

Her first instinct was to stop the practice entirely. If this was what self-compassion did, she did not want any more of it. She closed her notebook. She put the book away. She went to bed early.

The next morning she got curious. She had read something in the book about a phenomenon called backdraft. She went back to the chapter. The description matched what had happened to her, word for word. She had not broken anything. The practice had worked exactly as designed. She had just not been warned that "working" sometimes looked like a sobbing heap on the living room floor.

What she was about to learn was that the sobbing was not the end of the practice. It was the middle. And the practice only finishes working if you keep going through the middle, not around it.

What You'll Get From This Chapter

This chapter explains backdraft: the phenomenon where opening yourself to kindness brings up old pain. You will learn why this happens, why it is a sign the practice is working rather than failing, and how to work through it safely. You will see real examples of people who hit backdraft and what helped them move through it. You will also learn when backdraft crosses the line into something that needs professional support. By the end, you will have a working relationship with what is probably the most misunderstood experience in compassion practice.

16.1 What Backdraft Is

Backdraft is a term borrowed from firefighting. When a fire has been burning in a closed room and has used up most of the oxygen, opening the door can cause the sudden rush of fresh air to ignite a fireball. The flames come rushing out. What looks like a harmless act (opening a door) triggers an intense reaction.

Kristin Neff and Christopher Germer adopted the word for what happens in compassion practice. When you open the door to kindness, old pain sometimes comes rushing out. Grief you did not know you had. Anger you had been holding for years. Memories of unmet needs. The practice itself does not cause the pain. The pain was already there, sealed in a closed room of your psyche, and the warmth simply opened the door (Germer & Neff, 2013).

This is one of the most important things to understand about CFT practice. If you have a long history of not being cared for, or of being cared for badly, your body and mind have been holding the absence as a kind of quiet ache for a long time. When you start offering yourself what was missing, the contrast between what you now have and what you did not have becomes sharply visible. The ache, which had been mostly invisible, becomes visible. It hurts, because it was always hurting, and you had only stopped noticing.

The pain is not new. It is simply newly felt.

16.2 Why Kindness Can Trigger Grief

Several mechanisms produce backdraft. Understanding them will help you hold the experience when it happens.

Contrast. When you feel warmth now, your body, often for the first time, gets clear information about what warmth feels like. This makes the absence of warmth, in the past, suddenly real. You can only grieve what you can see you have lost. Kindness makes the losses visible.

Signal of safety. Your body, during the practice, is starting to feel safer than it usually does. When a body feels safer, it begins to release material it was holding because it was not safe enough to feel before. Tears. Shaking. Waves of emotion. This is called titration by some therapists. The body does its own titration when given the right conditions.

175

Attachment memory. The specific quality of being cared for, coming from an imagined compassionate other or from your own compassionate self, activates attachment-related memories. If your early attachment was disrupted, warmth can touch that old wound. The warmth is not creating the wound. The warmth is touching a wound that was already there (Mikulincer & Shaver, 2007).

Old defenses dissolving. Self-criticism is, among other things, a defense. It keeps you from feeling certain things. When self-compassion replaces self-criticism, the defense drops, and the feelings it was holding back come through. Some readers experience this as a flood. Others experience it as a slow leak over weeks.

None of this is pathology. All of it is the system doing what systems do when they begin to heal. The discomfort is not a sign that the practice is harmful. It is a sign that the practice is reaching something real.

16.3 A Real Example

Tomas had lost his mother when he was eleven. His father had remained, functionally, but emotionally absent. Tomas had been a self-sufficient child by necessity. He had grown into a self-sufficient adult. He did not ask for help. He did not lean on anyone. He was the kind of person his friends described as "so strong."

At forty-two, he started CFT therapy because his marriage was in trouble. His wife had told him she felt like she did not have a partner. She had been asking him, for years, to let her in. He did not know how.

Backdraft hit him in the fourth session. His therapist had guided him through a brief compassionate other practice. He had chosen his late mother as the figure. He had been a little worried about this choice. His therapist had checked in with him. He had said he was fine. He thought he was.

During the practice, he saw his mother. She was looking at him with the quiet, steady love he remembered from when he was small. She was saying, without words, that she was proud of him. That she had missed watching him grow up. That she was sorry she had not been there.

Tomas broke down in the therapist's office in a way he had not allowed himself to break down since he was eleven. He cried for twenty minutes. When he could speak again, he said, "I have been walking around for thirty-one years pretending I was fine. I have not been fine."

That was the beginning of something. Not the end. The grief that came up in that session took months to move through. He cried in his car. He cried in the shower. He cried at a gas station at 11 p.m. after hearing a song on the radio. The practice had opened a door that had been closed for three decades, and a lot of what had been behind the door needed to come out.

Six months later, his wife told him he had changed. She did not mean that he was suddenly different. She meant that he was suddenly present. He was letting her in. He was allowing himself to need her, and to be needed by her, in a way he had not been able to before. The grief had not ruined him. The grief had opened him.

What this means for you: Backdraft is often the entry point to material that was already there but could not come out until it had somewhere safe to land. The practice is the somewhere safe. If tears come, let them. They are not an interruption to the healing. They are part of it.

16.4 How To Work With It

When backdraft happens, your system is asking for specific things. Here is what actually helps.

Stop trying to fix it. Your instinct, especially if you are used to self-criticism, will be to solve the crying, calm the body down, get back to normal. Do not. Let the wave move through you. It has a shape. It rises, peaks, and falls. If you ride it, it will complete itself. If you fight it, it may last much longer.

Drop the deep practice. If you are in the middle of a guided practice and backdraft hits hard, you can stop the practice. Come back to the external world. Feel your feet on the floor. Notice five things you can see. Let your body return to the room. You do not have to finish the practice. The practice will still be available tomorrow.

Use physical grounding. A cool glass of water. A hand on your chest. A hand on your belly. The weight of a blanket. Your dog if you have one. The body is flooded. Giving it something concrete to touch helps it settle.

Move. After the wave has mostly passed, a short walk often helps. The body is asking to discharge. Walking, slowly, lets the nervous system integrate what just happened.

Do not practice again immediately. Give the system a day or two to digest. Go back to the simplest version of the practice (soothing rhythm breathing only) before returning to the more activating ones (compassionate other, letters). Build back up slowly.

Write about it later. When you are settled, write down what came up. Not to analyze. Just to witness. The writing tells the material that it was seen, and seen material is less likely to ambush you again.

If you have access to a therapist, this is a good time to bring what came up into a session. If you do not, move slower with the practices for a while and let the next wave teach you what it needs.

16.5 Another Real Example

Salma had complex feelings about her father. He had been critical, demanding, and emotionally unavailable throughout her childhood. He had also been her biggest advocate, the person who had pushed her to apply to the medical school she had eventually gotten into. She had never been able to reconcile the two versions of him.

She was trying the compassionate self practice one Sunday afternoon. She was in her living room. She was doing it by the book. Upright posture, soft face, slow breath, imagined wisdom and strength and warmth.

What came up was not grief. It was rage.

She was suddenly furious with her father. Not abstractly. Specifically. Scene after scene played in her mind of moments he had dismissed her, criticized her, refused to say the thing she had needed to hear. She had been a dutiful daughter for forty years, sending him money, calling on his birthday, arranging his medical care. She had never, once, allowed herself to be angry with him. Now she was.

She did not know what to do. The rage felt dangerous. Like if she opened that door further, she might never close it again. She might do something she would regret. She might call him and say things she could not take back.

She did something that turned out to be wise. She did not call him. She went to her kitchen. She got a pen and a notebook. She wrote for an hour. She wrote everything. Every grievance. Every moment of dismissal. Every sentence she had held back for forty years. The page filled. She kept writing.

When she was done, she closed the notebook. She did not send it to anyone. She sat with her hand on the cover for a long time.

Over the next two weeks, the rage softened. Not because she had solved it. Because she had let it speak. The rage had been part of what the self-criticism had been containing. She had been keeping herself small, in part, to avoid feeling the full force of what she felt about the people who had made her small.

Six months later, she was able to have a real conversation with her father, one in which she told him some of what she had been holding. It was not a reconciliation. It was an honest exchange. He did not apologize. He did something more surprising. He listened. For the first time in her life, he listened.

What this means for you: Backdraft does not always look like grief. Sometimes it looks like rage. Sometimes it looks like a wave of shame. Sometimes it looks like fear, dread, or confusion. Whatever shape it takes, the instructions are the same. Let it move. Do not act on it immediately. Witness it. Let it settle. Then, later, decide what, if anything, to do with what you have learned.

16.6 When It Is Time To Call For Help

Most backdraft is manageable with the tools in this chapter. Some is not. Here is how to tell the difference.

Manageable backdraft produces strong feelings that rise, peak, and fall within a session or a few hours. You feel wrung out afterward, but you feel more yourself, not less. You are able to function the next day. The material that came up feels significant but workable. You sleep that night.

Harder backdraft includes any of the following: Flashbacks that feel like the past is happening now, Dissociation (feeling outside your body, or that the world is not real), Intrusive memories that will not settle, Panic that does not pass within an hour, Thoughts of self-harm or suicide, and An inability to function for more than a day or two afterward.

If any of these show up, please work with a trauma-informed therapist before continuing with the deeper practices. This is not a failure. Some material is simply too big to process alone. A therapist can help you move through it with safety and pacing, and then the practice will be available to you again.

There is also a middle category. Some readers experience backdraft that is hard but not frightening. Strong grief that lasts a few days. Anger that takes a week to move through. Waves that come back for a month. This is often a sign that your system is metabolizing something real. Go slowly. Use the simpler practices (breathing, safe place) rather than the more activating ones (compassionate other, letters) while the digestion happens. Come back to the deeper practices when the waves have mostly settled.

16.7 Why This Is Worth It

Readers who hit backdraft often ask, at some point, if it is worth continuing. The practice is supposed to help. If the help hurts, why keep going?

The honest answer is that the hurt is not caused by the practice. The hurt is caused by what was already there. The practice is just the first time in your life that the pain had somewhere safe to be felt. If you stop the practice, the pain does not go away. It goes back to being invisible, sealed behind the old defenses. The defenses did not remove the pain. They just hid it. The practice is the first real opportunity for the pain to move, be seen, and eventually settle.

The alternative to backdraft is not painlessness. The alternative is a lifetime of the pain running your behavior from underneath, shaping your choices, keeping you small, tiring you out. Many readers, looking back after several months, say that the hard weeks of backdraft were some of the most important weeks of their lives. Not pleasant. Important.

You do not have to enjoy backdraft. You only have to be willing to move through it, at the pace your system can handle, with support where needed.

16.8 When It Doesn't Work

Some readers do everything in this chapter and still find backdraft overwhelming. Here is what to try.

If backdraft keeps flooding you. Slow down. Do one minute of breathing only. No imagery. No compassionate other. Just breath. For two weeks. Let your system recalibrate. Then try one minute of safe place. Build up from the smallest possible dose.

If you are afraid of the next wave. Fear of backdraft can become its own problem. You start avoiding practice because you do not want another flood. Two things to try. First, remind yourself that nothing you have experienced so far has damaged you; the waves have moved through. Second, practice only when you have an open afternoon. Not before a big day. Not before bed. Not before a social event. Give yourself permission to fall apart if you need to.

If you cannot tell if what you are feeling is backdraft or a crisis. Call someone. A therapist. A friend. A crisis line. When in doubt, get support. You do not have to diagnose yourself while you are in the middle of something hard.

If the practices feel completely unsafe. Put the book down. This is not a sign of weakness. Your nervous system is telling you it needs more foundation before it can do this work. Often that foundation is a therapist, stable sleep, medication if needed, social support, or a period of less intense practice. Come back to the book when the ground is firmer. The book will still be here.

16.9 Wrapping Up

Backdraft is the phenomenon where opening yourself to kindness brings up old pain. It is one of the most common and most misunderstood experiences in compassion practice. It is not a sign that the practice is broken. It is a sign that the practice has reached something real.

The pain is not new. It was already there. What is new is that you now have the conditions to feel it. That is good news, even when it does not feel like good news.

When backdraft happens, stop trying to fix it. Let the wave move. Use physical grounding. Slow down the practice for a few days. Write about what came up when you are settled. Come back to the deeper practices slowly. If the material is too big, get professional support. There is no failure in that.

Most backdraft is manageable with the tools in this chapter. Some is not. Know the signs that mean you need more support, and get it if you need it.

For this week, do not go looking for backdraft. Practice gently. If it comes, work with it using what you have learned. If it does not come, that is fine too. Some readers experience significant backdraft. Others experience almost none. The pace is individual. Follow yours.

In the next chapter, you will look at how your past, especially early attachment and trauma, shapes the practice. For some readers, that chapter will explain why this work has felt the way it has. For others, it will offer tools specific to their history.

Chapter 17: When Your Past Gets In The Way

Darius was thirty-six years old and he had never cried in front of another human being. Not as an adult. Not since he was about seven, when he had learned that crying in his house made things worse, not better. He had gotten very good at not crying. It was an accomplishment he had taken some quiet pride in for most of his life.

He had been doing the practices for two months. Soothing rhythm breathing was fine. Safe place was fine, once he had settled on the garage of the house he had bought at thirty, alone, the first space he had ever owned. The compassionate other was harder. No figure would stay in his mind for more than a few seconds. He kept trying.

His therapist asked him, in their third month together, a simple question. "When you were a child, when you were hurt or scared, who did you go to?"

Darius thought about it. He could not, at first, think of anyone. He searched. His father had been angry. His mother had been depressed and unavailable. His older brother had been cruel. His teachers had been indifferent. He had gone to no one. He had learned, very young, to go nowhere with his pain. Pain, in his system, was something to handle alone, in the dark, by muscle and will. There was no other option.

When he told his therapist this, she was quiet for a long time. She finally said, "You have been trying to do a practice that requires an internal model of being cared for. You do not have that model. It is not surprising you are struggling."

That sentence was a relief. Not because it solved anything. Because it named something he had not been able to name. He was not failing at the practice. The practice required something that had never been built in him, and the building was going to take longer than two months, and longer than a book, and possibly longer than a year of therapy. He was not broken. He was early.

What You'll Get From This Chapter

This chapter addresses what happens when your early history gets in the way of the practices. You will learn how attachment experiences shape your capacity for self-compassion, why trauma makes the work harder (but not impossible), how to adapt the practices for a nervous system that has been through significant harm, and when to seek professional support. By the end, you will have a clearer map of your own starting point and the tools to move at the right pace for your specific history.

17.1 Why Your Past Matters

Your capacity for self-compassion, like most emotional capacities, was largely shaped in the first few years of your life. The soothing system, the part of your nervous system that produces warmth and calm, develops through contact with caregivers who offered consistent, attuned care. When that contact was available, you developed an internal template for being soothed. When it was not, you did not (Bowlby, 1988; Cassidy & Shaver, 2016).

This is not destiny. It is starting point. People with difficult early histories can develop strong self-compassion as adults. It just takes longer, requires more repetition, and sometimes needs more help. If you have been finding the practices harder than the book seemed to promise they would be, your history may be why.

The main categories of early experience that shape self-compassion capacity are:

Secure attachment. Caregivers were mostly available, attuned, and responsive. You learned that your feelings mattered and that help was available. As an adult, you have a working internal model of care. Self-compassion comes more easily.

Anxious attachment. Caregivers were inconsistent. Sometimes available, sometimes not. You learned to work harder for care, to watch carefully for signals, to fear abandonment. As an adult, you may have a strong outward flow of compassion (you take care of others) but struggle to receive it or direct it inward.

Avoidant attachment. Caregivers were dismissive of emotional needs. You learned to deactivate your own needs, to be self-sufficient, to avoid asking for help. As an adult, the incoming and self-directed flows of compassion may be almost completely shut down. You can think about them but not feel them.

Disorganized attachment. Caregivers were a source of both care and fear. You learned that the people who were supposed to help you also hurt you. As an adult, compassion (from others or to yourself) may feel actively threatening, because it activates old contradictions.

If you do not know which category fits you, that is fine. You do not need a label. The point is to understand that your starting point is not the same as everyone else's, and the practice will feel different depending on where you started.

17.2 Trauma Changes The Work

Trauma is more specific than difficult attachment. Trauma is an experience, or a series of experiences, that overwhelmed your nervous system's capacity to process them. The system could not digest what happened. It stored the raw material, in the body and in specific networks of memory, and the material has been affecting your current experience ever since (van der Kolk, 2014).

When you have trauma, several things happen that make self-compassion harder.

Your threat system is calibrated high. You scan for danger more than other people. Softness can read as a setup. Kindness can feel like a trap. This is not a belief. It is a body state.

Certain practices can activate the trauma. Eyes closed. Slow breathing. Stillness. These conditions, which are calming for many, can be triggering for trauma survivors. The same conditions that let the parasympathetic system engage also let unprocessed material come closer to the surface.

Compassion can feel foreign or threatening. If the people who were supposed to love you hurt you, love itself becomes confusing. When someone offers you care, or when you try to offer it to yourself, the body can interpret it as a signal that something bad is about to happen, because that has been the historical pattern.

Dissociation can interfere. Many trauma survivors have developed the capacity to leave their bodies, mentally, when things get overwhelming. This served them in childhood. In adulthood, it can mean they cannot fully arrive in the practices, because they are not fully in their bodies.

None of this means the practice cannot work for you. It does mean that the practice may need to be modified, paced differently, or done alongside professional support. Generic instructions (close your eyes, breathe deeply, imagine a warm figure) can actually backfire for a trauma-sensitive nervous system. What follows are modifications that make the work safer and more effective.

17.3 A Real Example

Mei had been sexually abused by a family member between the ages of six and twelve. She had not told anyone until she was thirty-one. She had been in therapy for three years by the time she came across CFT. Her therapist had suggested it as a supplement to the trauma work they had been doing.

The first practice she tried was soothing rhythm breathing. It should have been the simplest. It sent her into a panic attack within ninety seconds. Slow breathing, with her eyes closed, had triggered something the therapist later identified as a somatic flashback. Her body had gone back, without her permission, to a moment of stillness and quiet that had preceded an assault.

She did not try the practice again for six weeks. She and her therapist worked on trauma processing. When she came back to the breathing, they made several modifications. She kept her eyes open, focused on a neutral object. She did the breathing for one minute, not five. She did it during the day, not at night. She added a warm drink in her hand as a physical anchor. She did it with her therapist in the room for the first several attempts.

It worked, slowly, with the modifications. A year later, she could do five minutes of soothing rhythm breathing with her eyes closed, in her own home, without activation. Not every day. But often enough that the practice became usable.

Her compassionate other was a small child version of herself. Her therapist had suggested this, with hesitation, because it is an unusual choice. For Mei, it worked. She could not tolerate a figure that might, in some way, resemble a caregiver. A younger version of herself felt safe because it was unambiguously on her side, and it carried no history of betrayal. She would imagine herself at seven, bringing that child into her adult safe place, and would offer her the care she wished someone had offered her at that age.

Over two years of combined work, Mei's relationship with the practices changed. They were not the solution to her trauma. They were part of the healing, alongside the trauma processing. She describes the combination as what finally let her feel something other than either numbness or terror.

What this means for you: If generic versions of the practices do not work for you, they can often be modified. Eyes open. Shorter duration. External grounding. A compassionate other that fits your specific history. A therapist in the room at first. The modifications are not cheating. They are the right version for a nervous system that has been through more than most.

17.4 Modifications That Help

Here is a working list of modifications to use if your history makes the standard practices hard.

For the breathing practice:

Keep your eyes open, focused on a neutral object (a candle, a plant, a corner of the room).

Start with one minute, not five. Add thirty seconds a week.

Do the practice in the morning or early afternoon, not at night.

Hold something warm (a mug of tea, a heated cloth) during the practice.

Sit with your back against a wall or a sturdy chair so you can feel a solid surface behind you.

If you start to feel activated, stop. Stand up. Move. Come back tomorrow.

For the safe place practice:

Let the place be small and contained, not vast and open. A cabin. A car. A closet. Open spaces can feel exposing.

Do not invite any human figures into the place, even briefly, until you feel stable in the place alone.

Add multiple exits to the place. Being trapped, even in imagination, can trigger some systems.

Make the place completely unlike any place associated with past harm.

For the compassionate other practice:

Non-human figures (animals, trees, beings of light) are often safer than human ones.

A younger version of yourself can work well if human caregivers feel dangerous.

Figures from fiction or mythology can work because they have no history with you.

The figure does not need to speak. Silent presence is often enough.

For letter writing:

Write in short segments. Five sentences. Not full pages.

Write about present-day situations, not past trauma, until you have done significant trauma work.

If material from the past starts to come up, close the notebook. Process it in therapy, not alone.

For chair work:

Do it first with a therapist, not alone, if your critic is connected to past harm.

The chair work can surface voices that are not just internal but carry the weight of specific people from your past. This is manageable in therapy. It can be destabilizing alone.

17.5 Another Real Example

Elijah was a veteran. He had served two combat tours and had come home with PTSD. He had been in treatment for four years before a therapist introduced him to CFT practices as an adjunct to his existing trauma work.

His first attempt at soothing rhythm breathing produced a flashback. He described it later as being back in the truck, minutes before the event that had nearly killed him and had killed two of his friends.

His therapist moved carefully. She did not abandon the practice. She adapted it. For the first three months, Elijah did the breathing standing up, with his eyes open, facing a window. Not sitting, not with his eyes closed. Standing, facing out. She framed it as "awareness breathing" rather than "soothing breathing," to sidestep the word "soothing," which his system did not yet trust.

His compassionate other was not a person or an animal. It was a mountain. An actual mountain he knew, from a hiking trip he had taken three summers ago. The mountain was ancient, steady, unmoved by human events. Elijah could hold the mountain in his mind without triggering anything. The mountain did not ask him to feel warmth, which his system still could not reliably produce. The mountain just was. Steady. Present. Real.

Over a year, his practice expanded. He eventually sat down. He eventually closed his eyes. He eventually let the mountain have a warmer quality in his imagination, like afternoon sun on a cliff face. He never chose a human figure. The mountain was enough.

He described the practice, two years in, as one of three things that had made the biggest difference in his recovery. The other two were the trauma therapy itself and a specific friendship with another veteran who had been in group with him. He did not present the practice as a miracle. He presented it as a quiet, reliable tool that had, with enough time and the right modifications, become his.

What this means for you: You do not have to force your practice to look like the practices in books. A veteran with PTSD does not need to pretend he can close his eyes and imagine a warm grandmother. A survivor of childhood abuse does not need to pretend her compassionate other is a wise elder. The practice belongs to you. The shape it takes for your specific system is the right shape, even if it does not match the examples.

17.6 Knowing When To Get Help

Some readers will be able to work with this book on their own. Many will need additional support. Here are signs that professional help would make a real difference.

You have a significant trauma history. Any of: childhood abuse or neglect, sexual assault, combat exposure, a major accident or medical trauma, prolonged domestic violence, or sustained early attachment disruption. If any of these apply, a trauma-informed therapist will help you make faster and safer progress than you can make alone.

The practices consistently destabilize you. If you are hitting backdraft, flashbacks, or dissociation regularly and cannot move through them, you need support. Not because you are failing. Because the material needs more than solo work can provide.

You have thoughts of harming yourself. Please reach out to a mental health professional. The practices are not a substitute for clinical care when the stakes are high.

You have a mental health diagnosis you are managing. Depression, anxiety disorders, bipolar disorder, eating disorders, substance use disorders, PTSD. The practices can complement treatment, but they are not a replacement for it. A clinician can help you use them in a way that supports your overall plan.

You feel stuck after months of practice. If you have done the work consistently for six months and nothing is moving, a therapist can help you find what is in the way. Sometimes the answer is small. Sometimes it is bigger. Either way, outside eyes help.

Getting help is not a failure. It is the most practical move you can make. Many of the readers who have gotten the most out of CFT did so in combination with therapy. The book is a foundation. Therapy is the structure that goes on top of it, when the foundation needs more than a book can hold.

17.7 When It Doesn't Work

Some readers, even with the modifications in this chapter, find the practice will not land. Here is what to consider.

If you cannot find any version of a compassionate other that feels safe. This is often a sign of extensive early attachment disruption. It is not a permanent condition. It often shifts with time, with trauma work, and with enough real-world experiences of being cared for by safe people. In the meantime, focus on the practices that do not require a figure (breathing, simple body awareness). The figure will come, eventually, when the ground is ready.

If every attempt at practice leads to dissociation. This is a signal to stop solo practice and work with a trauma therapist. Dissociation is not something to push through. It is information. Your system is telling you it needs different conditions.

If you feel worse over weeks, not better. Please talk to a therapist. Some material, once surfaced, needs ongoing containment until it can be processed. Without that, the surfacing can be destabilizing rather than healing.

If you have tried everything and the practice is not for you right now. That is allowed. Put the book on the shelf. Come back in a year, or two, or five. Some people find CFT is right for them at a specific moment in their lives and not at others. Your timing is your timing. The book will keep.

17.8 The Short Answer

Your past shapes your starting point. If your early attachment was disrupted, or if you experienced trauma, the standard versions of the practices will likely be harder for you, and sometimes counterproductive. This is not a sign that you cannot do the work. It is a sign that the work needs to be adapted for your specific system.

Modifications include eyes-open breathing, contained safe places, non-human compassionate figures, shorter practice durations, external grounding, and the use of neutral anchors rather than warm ones. Any or all of these can make the practices usable for a nervous system that has been through significant harm.

Some readers need professional support alongside the practices. If you have a significant trauma history, a mental health diagnosis, or thoughts of harming yourself, please get help. The practices can complement clinical care. They cannot replace it.

For this week, notice what is working and what is not. If something is consistently activating, change the conditions. Eyes open. Shorter duration. A different figure. Give yourself permission to modify. Your practice is yours. The right shape for you is the one you can actually sustain.

In the next chapter, you move into Part Six, which is about taking the practice off the page and into your daily life. The last three chapters address how compassion functions in your everyday activity, your relationships, and your continued growth. You have done substantial work to get here. Keep going.

PART VI: LIVING IT

Chapter 18: Compassion In Daily Life

Ibrahim was in his car on a Wednesday afternoon. The light had just turned red. He was two blocks from his kid's school and he was already four minutes late for pickup. His phone was buzzing. A coworker had sent a long email that needed a response by 5 p.m. He had not eaten lunch. He had a dinner to cook as soon as he got home because his wife was working late.

Under the old system, this moment would have produced a cascade. A tightness in his chest. A silent string of self-criticism. *You are always running late. You cannot manage your time. Your kid will be the last one there again. What kind of father cannot get to school on time.* He would arrive at the school in a worse mood than when he left, and his kid would feel it.

Today, something different happened. He noticed the chest tightness. He noticed the self-criticism about to start. He did three things in about ten seconds.

He took a slow breath. Long on the exhale.

He put his right hand on his chest, briefly, at the red light.

He said one sentence to himself, not out loud but clearly. "This is a hard moment. It is not a character flaw. It is a red light."

The light turned green. He drove the last two blocks. He arrived at the school about five minutes late, which was about the same as he had been on a dozen previous Wednesdays. His kid was fine. The coworker's email could wait an hour. Dinner would happen. He was not late because he was a bad father. He was late because traffic in that junction was bad on Wednesdays and he had been through three such junctions to get there.

The whole sequence had taken less than fifteen seconds. It had changed the character of the rest of his afternoon.

What You'll Get From This Chapter

This chapter is about taking the practices off the cushion and into the middle of your actual day. You will learn a set of brief, practical practices you can use in under a minute anywhere: at work, in traffic, between meetings, before bed, during hard conversations. You will see how to weave compassion into your routine without adding a single new thing to your schedule, and you will learn the specific moments when micro-practices produce the biggest shifts. By the end, you will have a practical, everyday version of the work that does not require a quiet room or a spare half hour.

18.1 The Real Test

The dedicated practices in Part Four are the foundation. They build the pathway. But the real test of compassion is not what you can do with twenty minutes in a quiet room. The real test is what happens in your car, in your kitchen, in the three-minute gap between meetings, when the kids are yelling, when the email arrives, when the dog throws up on the rug.

Most readers of self-help books do the exercises for a few weeks and expect their lives to transform. Life does not transform in a quiet room. Life transforms in the middle of itself. The book practices are there to train the skill. The skill gets used out in the world. If you never bring the skill out of the room, the training does not accumulate into anything that matters.

The good news is that the transfer from formal practice to daily life is easier than most readers think. You do not need to set aside new time. You do not need to change your schedule. You just need to attach small compassion practices to moments that were already happening. A deep breath at a red light. A hand on the chest in the bathroom mirror. A sentence of kindness to yourself in the elevator. These micro-practices, done consistently, produce more change than the formal sessions do on their own.

Formal practice builds the skill. Informal practice integrates it.

18.2 The Self-Compassion Break

The most useful micro-practice in the whole field of self-compassion work is a three-part sequence that takes about thirty seconds. Kristin Neff calls it the self-compassion break. Gilbert's version has a similar shape. You can use it any time you notice you are struggling (Neff & Germer, 2013).

The three parts are:

Step 1: Name what is happening. "This is a hard moment." Or "This is stress." Or "This is pain." Whatever fits. Naming the experience takes it out of the background and into awareness. The naming alone often produces a small settling.

Step 2: Recognize that this is part of being human. "Other people feel this too." Or "This is what it is like to be human." Or "I am not alone in this." The critic isolates you. The critic tells you that your struggle is uniquely your fault. Reminding yourself that struggle is a human experience breaks the isolation.

Step 3: Offer yourself kindness. "May I give myself what I need right now." Or "May I be gentle with myself in this moment." Or "This is hard, and I am here." A phrase of care, directed at yourself. You can pair it with a hand on your chest if you want.

That is the whole practice. Thirty seconds. Anywhere. At a red light. In a bathroom. On a walk. Before opening a difficult email.

During a hard conversation. The three steps can be done silently. No one will know you are doing it.

Readers often dismiss this practice as too simple. It is too simple for what you want it to do. Thirty seconds should not change much. But repeated thirty-second doses, multiple times a day, over months, change a nervous system more than one twenty-minute session a day. The drip matters more than the flood.

18.3 Anchors That Work

One of the fastest ways to make informal practice stick is to anchor it to things you were already going to do. You are not adding new activities. You are adding a micro-practice to existing ones. Some anchors that work well:

Walking through doorways. Every time you walk through a door, take one deep breath. Every time. Grocery store. Office. Bathroom. You walk through twenty doors a day. That is twenty breaths.

Waiting at red lights. Every red light is a chance to do a full slow-breath cycle or a self-compassion break. The practice works even with your eyes open on the road.

Hand on the faucet. Every time you turn on water (to wash hands, do dishes, start a shower), pause for one breath before you turn it on. One breath. You do this four or five times a day minimum.

Phone notifications. When your phone buzzes, use it as a micro-cue. One breath. Name one thing you are feeling. Then decide if you want to look at the notification.

Before meals. Ten seconds before eating. Hand on the belly. One phrase of thanks, to yourself or to whatever you find thankable.

At bedtime. Before you turn out the light, one minute of slow breathing and one kind sentence to yourself about the day.

Pick one anchor. Not six. One. Do it for two weeks. Then add another. Anchors that stick are the ones that become automatic. Anchors that do not stick are usually ones that required you to remember on your own. Remembering is expensive. Attaching is cheap.

18.4 A Real Example

Celeste is a high school teacher. She has 160 students across five classes. She eats her lunch standing up, at her desk, in 22 minutes. She does not have a quiet room at school. She does not have a quiet room at home either, because she has three kids and one bathroom.

She tried formal CFT practice for about six weeks. It did not stick. She would intend to sit down for ten minutes in the evening. Something would come up. A kid would need help with homework. Laundry would need folding. She was exhausted. By the time the house was quiet at 10 p.m., she did not have ten minutes of attention left for anything.

Her therapist suggested, almost offhand, that she try skipping the formal practice for a month and doing only micro-practices. Celeste was skeptical. She had read enough to believe the formal sessions were the real work.

She tried it anyway. She picked two anchors. Every time she walked through the classroom door, she took one slow breath. Every time she turned on the car, she put her hand on her chest for three seconds and said, silently, "I am doing my best today."

That was it. Two anchors. Each one took less than ten seconds. She used each one, on average, about six or seven times a day. By the end of the first week, she had done more than a hundred micro-practices. She did not feel dramatically different. But she felt, by Friday, a little less shredded than usual.

By week three, she had noticed something strange. She was slightly less reactive with her students. When a kid pushed back on an assignment, she did not go into full critic mode about her own teaching. She just noticed and responded. Her shoulders were lower. Her jaw was looser. She was not doing any more practice than she had been doing. The practice was just, finally, in the right container for her life.

Two months in, she added a third anchor. Before bed, one minute of breathing. That was the most she ever did. No formal forty-minute sessions. No meditation retreat. Three anchors, thirty seconds each, done dozens of times a day.

Her therapist pointed out, at six months, that the shifts she was seeing were as substantial as those in clients doing thirty-minute daily sessions. The medium had changed. The work was the same.

What this means for you: If the formal practice is not fitting your life, do not conclude that the work is not for you. Shift the container. Micro-practices, attached to things you were already doing, done many times a day, produce real change. Possibly more change than the formal sessions, because they reach more of your day.

18.5 Moments That Matter Most

Some moments in a day are more leveraged than others for compassion practice. If you can insert a practice at one of these moments, the effect is amplified. Key high-leverage moments:

The transition from work to home. Most people carry work stress into their evening without realizing it. A three-minute practice between leaving work and walking in the door of your house changes the next three hours of your life. This can be done in your car, on a walk, or standing on your own porch for one minute before you open the door.

Before a hard conversation. Thirty seconds of slow breathing and one kind sentence before you speak to someone difficult shifts the quality of the conversation substantially. Your voice is calmer. Your body is less defensive. You hear more of what the other person is saying.

After a hard conversation. Whatever just happened, some version of backdraft is coming. Give yourself thirty seconds. Hand on chest. "That was hard. It makes sense that I am shaken." This prevents the conversation from echoing through the rest of the day.

In the middle of the night. Many people wake between 2 and 4 a.m. with a racing mind. The critic is often loudest at that hour. A brief self-compassion break, with eyes closed, can put you back to sleep. It works better than trying to fight the thoughts.

When you catch yourself in critic mode. The moment you notice the critic speaking is a leveraged moment. Do not argue. Do not obey. Name what is happening. "The critic is loud." Three slow breaths. One compassionate sentence. The critic does not stop, but you get to choose your response, and the choice itself weakens the critic's power over time.

You do not need to use all of these. Pick one or two that correspond to moments that already hurt. Insert the practice at that point. Watch what happens.

18.6 Another Real Example

Rohan had developed a habit over twenty years of checking his email before he got out of bed in the morning. Within sixty seconds of opening his eyes, his heart rate was elevated, his jaw was clenched, and his day had already shifted into threat mode. His partner had told him, repeatedly, that he was "stressed before he even got up." Rohan had agreed. He had tried not checking email in the morning. He had failed every time.

His therapist suggested a compromise. He could check email. But he would add one thing first. Before his hand reached for the phone, he would put both hands on his chest for one breath and say, silently, "Whatever is in there, I can handle it, and I do not have to handle it instantly."

Rohan tried it. The first morning, he forgot. The second morning, he remembered halfway to the phone. The third morning, he did it before he touched the phone. By the end of two weeks, it had become automatic. The phone was still there. The emails were still there. But there was now a seven-second buffer between waking up and threat mode, and the buffer changed everything.

Six months later, Rohan's partner told him he was less tense in the mornings. Rohan had not told her about the new practice. She had noticed on her own. The micro-intervention had propagated out into the texture of his early mornings, and she had felt the difference without being able to name it.

He had not stopped checking email. He had not changed his job. He had not added meditation to his schedule. He had added seven seconds. Over months, the seven seconds had compounded.

What this means for you: Very small interventions, applied at the right moment, compound. You do not need to overhaul your life. You need to insert brief practices at the hinge points where your state tends to shift for the worse. Seven seconds of practice at the right moment is worth more than twenty minutes of practice at the wrong one.

18.7 When It Doesn't Work

Informal practice has its own failure modes. Here are the common ones.

You keep forgetting. This is the most common problem. The anchor was supposed to be automatic, and it is not. Two fixes. First, reduce the number of anchors to one. You probably picked too many. Second, attach the anchor to something physical you cannot miss. Not "every time I feel stressed" (you will miss many) but "every time I wash my hands" (you will not miss any). Physical cues beat emotional cues.

The practice feels forced. You are doing it, but it feels mechanical, like a performance. This is fine. Mechanical practice still works. The nervous system responds to the pattern, not to the sincerity. Over weeks, the mechanical quality softens into something more natural.

You feel silly doing it in public. You can do all of this silently, invisibly, without moving your face. No one needs to know. If you feel silly anyway, that is the critic. Name it. Keep practicing.

The critic hijacks the practice. You try to say a kind phrase to yourself and the critic says, "You do not deserve that." When this happens, you can switch to a neutral phrase. "This is a moment of stress." No kindness required. Just observation. The critic cannot argue with observation. The observation alone creates space, and the kindness will come later, once the ground has settled.

Nothing seems to be changing. The effects of informal practice are often gradual and invisible to you while they are happening. Ask someone close to you, after six weeks, if they have noticed anything. The people around you often see the changes before you do. If no one has noticed and you have not felt anything after three months, consider combining informal practice with some of the formal practices from Part Four. You may need both to get traction.

18.8 The Big Picture

The formal practices in Part Four build the skill. The informal practices in this chapter integrate the skill into your daily life. You need both. Formal alone tends to stay on the cushion. Informal alone never gets deep enough. Together, they produce real change.

Micro-practices work because they happen many times a day. Thirty seconds of practice, repeated fifteen times a day, is seven and a half minutes of practice across your day, but more importantly, it is distributed across all the moments that actually matter. A red light, a doorway, a hand on a faucet. These small moments accumulate into a different nervous system.

Anchor your practices to things you were already going to do. One or two anchors. Not six. Do them for two weeks before adding anything. The anchors that stick are the ones that become invisible. The anchors that fade were usually doing too much.

Focus on high-leverage moments. The transition from work to home. Before and after hard conversations. In the middle of the night. When you catch the critic speaking. Small interventions at these hinge points produce disproportionate change.

For this week, pick one anchor. Attach one micro-practice to it. Do it every time. Do not count. Do not grade. Just do it. Next week, you can add another. Or you can keep it at one. Both are fine.

In the next chapter, you will look at how compassion functions in your relationships. The flow toward others, the flow from others, and how the inward work changes both.

Chapter 19: Compassion In Relationships

Naomi had been married to Farid for eleven years. They had two kids, a house, and a list of ongoing arguments that had been running, in more or less the same form, for most of that time. The arguments were about chores, parenting styles, money, and in-laws. They had been to couples therapy twice. The therapy had helped for a few months each time, then faded.

This argument was about dishes. It was always about dishes. Farid had left his dishes in the sink again. Naomi had found them at 10 p.m., after she had already cleaned the kitchen once. She had felt the familiar surge. Her chest tightened. Her jaw clenched. A speech began composing itself in her head, a speech she had given a hundred times.

She was about to go into the bedroom and deliver it when she stopped in the hallway. She was not sure why. Something she had been working on for the last few months made her pause.

She took a slow breath. She noticed her body. Chest tight, jaw tight, hands clenched. She put her hand briefly on her chest. She asked herself, without planning to, a question she had been learning to ask. "What am I actually feeling?"

The answer that came was not what she expected. She was not angry about the dishes. She was lonely. She had been carrying the household for what felt like the entire marriage. The dishes were a reminder. Every dish in the sink was a small sentence that said she was alone in this. She had not felt seen or supported in a long time. The rage was a cover for a much older sadness.

She stood in the hallway for another minute. She did not go into the bedroom to fight. She went to the kitchen, loaded the dishes into the dishwasher (three minutes of actual work), and poured herself a glass of water. She sat at the kitchen table.

She went into the bedroom ten minutes later. She did not open with dishes. She said to her husband, "I feel really lonely. I have for a long time. I do not know how to change it, but I need you to know."

He put his book down. For the first time in maybe five years, they had a real conversation that night. Not a fight. A conversation. The dishes never came up. They talked until midnight. She cried. He apologized for things that had nothing to do with dishes. They went to sleep holding hands, which they had not done in months.

The argument had not been about dishes. The argument had never been about dishes. The practice of self-compassion had let her, for the first time in eleven years, catch what was actually going on in her own body before she exported it.

What You'll Get From This Chapter

This chapter addresses how compassion functions in relationships. You will learn how the inner work changes the way you speak to the people in your life, how to handle difficult family members without losing yourself, how to repair after rupture, and why limits are a form of compassion, not a failure of it. By the end, you will have a working framework for bringing the three flows of compassion (to self, to others, from others) into balance in the relationships that matter most to you.

19.1 The Inside Out Effect

The most reliable way to change your relationships is not to work on communication techniques. It is to change what is happening inside you before you speak.

Most relationship conflict is not caused by the surface issue. It is caused by unprocessed emotion from inside the person who is speaking. If you are operating from threat, your voice will sound like threat, no matter how carefully you phrase your sentences. If you are operating from shame, your partner will hear shame, even if you think you are hiding it. If you are operating from the compassionate self, your voice carries a quality people can feel, even without knowing why.

This is why self-compassion work has such a surprising effect on relationships. Readers often find, several months in, that their partners, kids, or friends say some version of "you seem different lately" without being able to specify what has changed. Usually, what has changed is that the reader is speaking from a different internal state. The words may be similar. The tone underneath the words has shifted.

This is also why communication techniques, by themselves, often fail. If you are still internally in threat mode, no amount of "I statements" will make the conversation go well. The nervous system of the other person is reading your nervous system, and your nervous system is still saying danger. The technique is a cosmetic layer over a biological transmission.

The inside-out effect means you do not have to master new conversational skills to improve your relationships. You have to become, slightly, a different kind of person on the inside. That work is the compassion work. The relationships change as a side effect of the inside shifting.

19.2 The Pause

The single most useful relational skill from this work is the pause. The small break between what someone says or does and what you say or do in response.

Most relational damage happens in the instant of reaction. A comment lands. Your body surges. You react, fast, without processing. The reaction is usually an amplified version of what the other person did, which invites them to amplify further, and the escalation is underway within thirty seconds. By the time either of you tries to stop the escalation, the conversation is already in a place neither of you wanted.

The pause is simple and hard. When something triggers you, you wait before responding. The wait does not have to be long. Three seconds. Sometimes two. During the pause, you do something internal. A breath. A hand on your chest. A quick question to yourself. "What am I actually feeling?" Then you respond.

The response that comes after a pause is almost always different from the response that would have come without the pause. It is more honest. It is less sharp. It matches what is actually happening rather than the first threat-driven version of what is happening.

The pause is a practice. You will miss it most of the time for the first several months. That is fine. Each time you catch a pause, the pathway strengthens. Over a year, you will catch maybe half your reactions before they fire, which is enough to change the texture of every important relationship in your life.

19.3 A Real Example

Gabi had a difficult relationship with her mother. Every phone call produced the same pattern. Her mother would say something critical, subtle but cutting. Gabi would flare. They would have a three-minute fight. They would both say things they did not mean. They would hang up angry. Gabi would spend the rest of the evening stewing. Her mother would call her sister to complain about her. The cycle had been running for twenty years.

Gabi started working on the pause during CFT therapy. She made a deal with herself. Before she responded to anything her mother said on the phone, she would take one slow breath. That was it. One breath. She would not try to be wiser, kinder, or more mature. She would just breathe once.

The first call after this commitment went badly. Her mother said something cutting within ninety seconds. Gabi reacted immediately, without breathing. The fight happened as usual. Gabi hung up annoyed at herself. She had not done the pause.

The second call, she managed one breath out of three provocations. The provocation where she paused turned out differently than the other two. Her response was flat rather than sharp. Her mother, not getting the expected flare, moved on to a different topic. Gabi noticed.

Over six months, Gabi got better at the pause. By month four, she was catching most of her reactions. The calls did not become warm. Her mother was still her mother. But the fights got shorter, less frequent, and less explosive. Gabi stopped dreading the calls.

At month six, something else happened. Her mother said something cutting. Gabi paused. She noticed, during the pause, that her mother sounded tired. Not mean. Tired. The comment had a quality of being said by someone who was not doing well. Gabi, from the pause, asked her mother, "Are you okay, Mom? You sound worn out." Her mother started crying. They had a real conversation for the first time in a decade. The critical comment had been a symptom of her mother's own struggle, not an attack on Gabi, and the pause had let Gabi see that.

The relationship with her mother did not become easy. But something substantive had shifted. Gabi had found, by pausing, that she could choose what to receive. The comments that were mean got much less response. The comments that were symptoms of her mother's pain got a different kind of response. She had become, in that relationship, a person who was not automatically hooked by every barb.

What this means for you: The pause is small and produces disproportionate change. It does not make difficult people less difficult. It makes you less reactive to them. The distance that opens in that two-second pause is enough to change what you are able to see and how you are able to respond.

19.4 Repair

Every relationship has rupture. This is not a failure. It is a feature. Humans are imperfect. Even skilled couples, close siblings, and best friends hurt each other regularly. What distinguishes healthy relationships from unhealthy ones is not the absence of rupture. It is the presence of repair (Gottman & Silver, 2015).

Repair is the process of acknowledging that something went wrong, taking responsibility for your part, and reconnecting. Most relationships fail not because the ruptures were too bad, but because the repairs did not happen, or happened too late.

Self-compassion makes repair easier. Here is why. Most people do not repair because repair requires acknowledging that they made a mistake. For a self-critical person, acknowledging a mistake activates the critic. The critic, which hates exposure, then makes repair feel unbearable. So the person defends instead of repairs. The rupture calcifies. The relationship erodes.

When you have built self-compassion, you can acknowledge mistakes without triggering the critic as hard. You can say, "I was short with you. I am sorry. I was stressed, and I took it out on you, and that was not fair." Saying this does not require you to collapse. You can admit the error and still be whole. That is what self-compassion makes possible. It gives you the ground to stand on while you apologize.

A useful structure for repair:

Acknowledge what you did. Specifically. Not "I am sorry for what happened." That is not a repair. That is a deflection. "I am sorry that I interrupted you three times tonight." That is a repair.

Own your part without over-explaining. You do not need to justify or contextualize. A brief explanation is fine. A long one turns the apology into a defense.

Acknowledge the impact. "I can see that it hurt you." Or "I can see that it made you feel dismissed." This step is the one most apologies skip. It is also the one that most matters.

Commit to something specific. Not "I will try to do better." That is too vague to help. "Next time I notice myself interrupting, I will stop and listen." Specific. Measurable.

Do not demand forgiveness. Repair is one-sided. You make the repair. The other person decides what to do with it. If you require them to forgive you immediately, your repair was really a request, and that is a different move.

19.5 Another Real Example

Farid, Naomi's husband from the opening, started his own work about a year after that hallway conversation. He had been defensive for most of their marriage, which he had always rationalized as reasonable. He had come home tired from work.

He had done his share. If Naomi was carrying more, it was because she wanted to, or because her standards were too high, or because she would not delegate.

In therapy, he started to see what he had been doing. He was using threat-system defenses. When Naomi criticized him, he counter-attacked or withdrew. He never, in eleven years of marriage, had simply said, "You are right. I dropped the ball." He had not been able to.

He started practicing, in small situations at work first. When a colleague pointed out a mistake he had made, instead of defending, he said, "You are right. I missed that. I will fix it." He reported to his therapist that the sentences felt physically hard to say. His chest tightened. His jaw clenched. But he said them, and the colleague moved on, and nothing bad happened.

He took the practice home. The first real repair with Naomi was about a forgotten anniversary. He had forgotten. He had, in past years, responded to this by explaining why he had forgotten, who was really at fault (usually his work schedule), and how Naomi was overreacting. This time, he stopped himself. He said, "I forgot our anniversary. I am sorry. It matters, and I am going to set reminders so this does not happen again."

Naomi was quiet for a long time. She finally said, "You have never said that to me." He said, "I know." They ended up having dinner out the following Saturday, at a restaurant he had booked that afternoon. They laughed during dinner for the first time in months.

The repair did not solve their marriage. They had more repairs to make, from both sides. But the capacity to repair had changed the whole arc. The ruptures that used to calcify were now more likely to close. And a marriage in which ruptures close is a different thing from one in which they accumulate.

What this means for you: Repair is a skill. Most people are not good at it because their threat system kicks in when they try. Self-compassion gives you the ground to repair from. The ability to say, simply, "I was wrong. I am sorry," without defending, changes the shape of every relationship that has been hurt by old ruptures.

19.6 Limits Are Compassion

Many readers confuse compassion with endless tolerance. They think that if they are becoming more compassionate, they must also become more forgiving, more available, more willing to put others first. This is a misunderstanding.

Real compassion, including self-compassion, includes limits. A parent who cannot say no to a child is not more compassionate than a parent who can. A friend who tolerates abusive behavior is not more compassionate than a friend who ends the relationship. A partner who accepts every betrayal is not more compassionate than one who enforces a limit.

Limits are compassion directed inward, so that you can continue to function as a caring person. Without limits, compassion collapses into burnout, resentment, or self-abandonment. A limit is the sentence, "I care about you, and I am not available for this." The two halves of the sentence belong together (Brown, 2018).

This is especially important in relationships with difficult family members, patterns from your family of origin, or partners who have been hurting you. Self-compassion does not require you to stay. It does not require you to tolerate more. It often requires the opposite. You may find, as you develop self-compassion, that you are less willing to tolerate things you used to tolerate. This is not a sign that the compassion has gone wrong. It is a sign that the compassion is including you.

Some limits you may find yourself needing: Shorter phone calls with a critical parent, An end to a conversation when a partner becomes abusive, A pause on visits with an in-law who speaks cruelly to you, A change in who handles a recurring family task, A slow distancing from a friendship that has become depleting, and A complete ending of a relationship that has been harmful.

None of these are easy. All of them, done from the compassionate self rather than from reactivity, can be done with clarity and without cruelty. You can love someone and not be available to them. The two things are not in conflict, even though the critic may tell you they are.

19.7 When It Doesn't Work

Compassion in relationships has its own failure modes. The common ones.

The other person does not reciprocate. You have been pausing, repairing, speaking from a calmer place. The other person is still doing exactly what they have always done. This is discouraging. It does not mean your work is useless. It means the relationship may have structural problems that self-compassion alone cannot solve. Your work is still working (in you). What happens between you and the other person depends on them too. Consider couples therapy, mediation, or a reassessment of the relationship.

You slip back into old patterns. You will. Regularly. The old patterns are older than the new ones. They will return under stress, when tired, when activated. Notice. Repair if needed. Start again.

The practice is not about never slipping. It is about the gradual lengthening of the stretches between slips.

You are accused of being cold. A family member, partner, or friend may tell you that you have become distant or unfeeling as you develop limits. This is common. For people who benefited from your previous over-giving, limits feel like coldness. Notice if the accusation is coming from someone who was taking advantage, or from someone you have actually hurt. The two situations need different responses.

You want to use the work to change the other person. It will not. The work changes you. The work may, indirectly, affect the other person, because they are responding to a different version of you. But you cannot practice self-compassion in order to make someone else different. That is a transaction, not a practice, and it usually fails.

You feel grief as you see old patterns clearly. This is normal and expected. Seeing what a relationship has been for years, without the filters, can produce grief. Grief for time lost. Grief for what might have been. Let the grief come. It is part of growing. It is not a sign that you should go back.

19.8 What To Remember

Your relationships change as you change. The most reliable way to shift a difficult relationship is not to master new communication techniques. It is to become, slightly, a different kind of person on the inside. That work is the compassion work. The relationships shift as a side effect.

The pause is the single most useful relational skill from this work. Two to three seconds between trigger and response. During the pause, a breath, a hand on the chest, or a quick internal question. The response after the pause is almost always different from the response that would have come without it.

Repair is a skill most people are not good at because their threat system fires when they try. Self-compassion gives you the ground to repair from. A clear, specific acknowledgment of what you did, ownership without over-explaining, recognition of the impact, and a specific commitment. Without a demand that the other person forgive you. That is repair.

Limits are compassion, not a failure of it. Saying "I care about you and I am not available for this" is one of the most loving sentences in the human vocabulary. It keeps you able to care over time. Without limits, compassion collapses. With them, it lasts.

For this week, pick one relationship where something has been hurting. Try the pause before your next difficult interaction. If a repair is available, try one. If a limit is needed, consider it. Small moves. Let the changes accumulate.

In the final chapter, you will look at where you go from here. What to expect over the next six months, the next year, the next five years. Resources for continued growth. And what this work looks like as it matures into something that shapes a whole life.

Chapter 20: Where You Go from Here

Sanjana finished reading this book on a Sunday evening, sitting on her couch with a cup of tea going cold next to her. She closed the book. She sat for a moment. She did not feel transformed. She did not feel like a different person. She felt, mostly, a little tired, a little tender, and quietly hopeful.

She thought about what she had learned. The three circles. The tricky brain. Her inner critic, which she could now name without flinching. The firefighter as the real shape of compassion. The compassionate self, which she had met a few times in practice. The soothing rhythm breathing, which she had been doing most evenings. Safe place imagery, which had been harder than she expected. Letters to herself, some of which had made her cry. The chair dialogue she had done once, awkwardly, in her living room.

She had not mastered any of it. Some of the chapters had been hard. A couple had produced nothing at all the first time through. She knew, closing the book, that this was not the end. It was something more like a map she now had, of a place she had just started to visit. The question was what she would do with the map.

She thought about her life a year from now. She could see, faintly, a version of herself who did these practices regularly, who was gentler with herself when things went wrong, who had harder conversations without destroying herself afterward. She could not promise that version of herself would appear. She could only commit to keep practicing, slowly, imperfectly, for long enough to find out.

She put the book on the shelf next to her bed. She made a note on her phone. "Practice tomorrow." She turned out the light.

What You'll Get From This Chapter

This chapter is about the long arc. You will see what realistic progress looks like over six months, a year, and five years of CFT practice. You will get a frame for the inevitable slumps, the unexpected returns of old patterns, and the moments when it seems nothing is working. You will learn about resources for continued learning, how to know when you need a therapist, and what it looks like when this work becomes a stable part of how you live. By the end, you will have a map for the years ahead, not just the next week.

20.1 What Progress Actually Looks Like

Progress in CFT is not linear. It is not a steady climb from the start to a destination. It looks more like a long, gentle upward trend with significant wobbles. Some weeks you feel you are moving forward. Some weeks you feel you have lost everything you gained. Some months you forget about the practices entirely. Some months you return to them with more conviction than ever.

This is normal. It is also the pattern in almost every long-term practice, from learning an instrument to building a friendship to recovering from illness. The steady-climb version does not exist. The wobbly-climb version is the real thing.

Here is a rough map of what readers typically report over the long arc.

At three months. You have some practices that work, at least some of the time. You have noticed the critic more often, though you still mostly obey it. You have had at least one or two moments that genuinely moved you. You have had plenty of sessions that produced nothing. You sometimes wonder if the whole thing is working.

At six months. Some of the practices have become automatic at small moments. Micro-practices. A breath at a red light. A hand on the chest before hard things. You have caught the critic in action several times and chosen a different response. You have had at least one significant backdraft wave, or you have experienced a smaller version multiple times. You are less reactive than you were.

At one year. The work has shaped several parts of your life, sometimes without you noticing. People close to you may have noticed changes. The critic still speaks, sometimes loudly, but you do not believe every word it says the way you used to. Your daily life has more small moments of warmth, which accumulate.

At three to five years. The practices have become part of who you are. You do not think of yourself as someone who "does CFT." You think of yourself as someone who tends to pause when triggered, who tends to name what is happening before reacting, who tends to speak to yourself with something closer to care than to contempt. The shift has been gradual enough that you may not fully see it, but it is substantial.

Your specific arc will look different from this. Some readers move faster. Some move slower. Some people make big leaps in month two and then plateau for a year. Some see almost nothing for six months and then, suddenly, a lot. The pace is individual. The direction is what matters.

20.2 The Slumps

Every long-term practice has slumps. Stretches where the practice stops working, feels empty, or gets abandoned. Slumps are not failure. Slumps are information.

Some common kinds:

The boredom slump. The practice has become routine. You are doing it, but nothing is happening anymore. You wonder if you have outgrown it. Usually, you have not. You have just reached a plateau. The plateaus are often where the deepest integration happens, underneath the surface. Keep practicing. Vary the form (different safe place, different figure, different time of day). The next phase will come.

The life-overload slump. Something has happened (a move, a baby, a death, a health crisis, a work crunch) and the practice has fallen away. You feel guilty. The guilt adds to the overload. Let the practice fall away for a while. Do micro-practices only. One breath at a red light. That is enough for now. When life has room again, the practice will return. Do not punish yourself for a life that got in the way.

The backdraft slump. You had a hard wave of old material. You have been avoiding the practice because you do not want another wave. Gently, slowly, come back. Start with the breath. Skip the more activating practices for a while. Let your system feel that the practice can be safe again.

The crisis slump. Something real is happening in your life, and the practices feel insufficient. You are probably right. Practices are not a substitute for getting help. If you are in a crisis, call a therapist, a crisis line, or a trusted person. Come back to the practice when the crisis has more footing.

The nothing-is-working slump. You have done everything in this book for a year and you feel like you have not changed. This is worth investigating. Is the practice reaching something real but producing changes you are not seeing because you are too close? Ask someone who knows you. Or is the practice, for some reason, not landing, and you need different help? A therapist can usually help you figure out which is which.

Slumps are part of the deal. Almost no one practices in a straight line. What matters is that you know slumps are normal and that you know how to return. Returning is more important than never leaving.

20.3 A Real Example

Ezra had done the practices for about ten months when he hit a wall. He had been doing everything right. Daily breathing, weekly letters, regular chair work. Things had been improving. Then, in month eleven, everything stopped working.

He would sit down to practice. Nothing would come. The compassionate other, who had been reliable for months, felt fake again. The letters felt like obligations. He noticed himself getting shorter with his partner, more reactive at work. He started avoiding practice altogether. A week became two weeks. Two weeks became a month.

He came into therapy feeling defeated. He told his therapist he thought the whole thing had stopped working, and that he was probably going to have to go back on the medication he had tapered off three months earlier.

His therapist asked him what had been happening in his life. Ezra listed things: his mother had fallen and was in rehab, his job had restructured, his kid had started high school, he had not slept well in weeks.

His therapist smiled gently. "Ezra. You are not having a practice problem. You are having a life problem. You have been handling a lot at once. No practice works in isolation from life. What you are experiencing is exactly what the system does when too much is happening at once."

She helped him design what she called a slump protocol. For the next month, he would do only micro-practices. One breath at a red light. One hand on his chest before hard things. No formal sessions. No letters. Just the micro-doses, multiple times a day. The formal practice would return when life settled.

He did it. For six weeks, that was his whole practice. By week four, he was less reactive. By week six, his mother was out of rehab and stable. He went back to formal practice. It worked again. The slump had not been a sign that the practice had stopped. It had been a sign that he had been over-loaded, and the over-loading had been interfering with the practice.

A year later, he looked back at that stretch as one of the most instructive months of his CFT journey. He had learned that the practice did not require perfect conditions. He had learned that micro-doses could carry him through a hard stretch. He had learned that returning after a slump was not starting over. It was resuming.

What this means for you: Slumps will come. The job is not to prevent them. The job is to know that they are normal, to adjust what you are doing without abandoning the practice entirely, and to return when life has room. Returning is not starting from zero. The pathways you have built are still there.

20.4 When To Get A Therapist

Some readers will do well with just this book. Many will not. This is not a reflection of your effort or your intelligence. It is a reflection of the fact that some material is too big for a book to hold, and some nervous systems need a human in the room to do this work safely.

Consider finding a therapist, especially one trained in CFT or compassion-focused work, if any of the following are true.

You have a significant trauma history, processed or not. The practices in this book touch material that trauma therapy can hold more safely.

You have a current mental health diagnosis that is not stable. The practices are not a substitute for treatment. A therapist can help you use them in a way that supports your overall plan.

You are finding backdraft or dissociation consistently overwhelming. These are not signs to push harder. They are signs to have help.

You have been practicing for six months and feel genuinely stuck, in a way that does not match the slump patterns above. A therapist can help you see what the book cannot.

You have thoughts of harming yourself. Please reach out to a mental health professional or a crisis line. This is not a book-level problem.

You are ready to go deeper than a book can go. A therapist can take the work places a book cannot, especially into the specific stories of your life.

Getting help is a sign of maturity, not a sign of failure. Many readers who have gotten the most from CFT did so in combination with therapy. The book is the foundation. The therapy is the architecture that goes on top. Together they hold more than either can hold alone.

20.5 What To Keep Doing

Here is a realistic, sustainable practice to aim for if you want the work to keep deepening over years.

Daily. Some version of soothing rhythm breathing. Can be as short as one minute. Can be scattered across the day as micro-practices rather than done in one sitting. The daily contact with the breath is the baseline that keeps everything else available.

Weekly. One longer session. Twenty to forty minutes, once a week. You can vary the practice: safe place one week, compassionate other another, chair work a third, letter writing a fourth. The longer session keeps the deeper pathways active.

Monthly. A check-in with yourself. Ten minutes to notice what has been working, what has fallen away, what is coming up. You can write this down. The monthly check-in keeps the practice from drifting without you noticing.

Occasionally. Read about compassion from a new angle. A book. A podcast. A talk. Fresh inputs keep the practice from going stale. Kristin Neff, Chris Germer, Paul Gilbert, and Chris Irons are all worth reading. So are writers outside the CFT tradition who write about care, kindness, and grief.

Always. Micro-practices. Breaths at red lights. Hands on chests before hard things. Pauses between triggers and responses. These cost almost nothing and accumulate into a changed nervous system over years.

You do not need to hit all of these every week. A good year is one where you did most of this, most of the time, with the usual slumps along the way. A perfect year is not the goal. The goal is a practice you can sustain, over decades, at a pace your life can hold.

20.6 Another Real Example

Rafael is sixty-seven. He started CFT therapy at fifty-one, after his first heart attack. He had been a classic self-critical man for the first half of his life. Military family. Hard father. A career in finance that had rewarded hardness. He had always thought self-compassion was for weaker people than him.

His cardiologist had suggested therapy. His therapist had, eventually, suggested CFT. He had been reluctant. He had tried it because he was running out of options for fixing the internal state that, his doctor had told him, was probably going to kill him before his genetics did.

The first two years had been hard. The practices felt foreign. The critic had attacked the work directly. He had almost quit several times. His therapist had kept showing up, patient and steady, not forcing, not demanding.

He had, slowly, learned. The breath. The safe place (a fishing spot he had loved as a child). The compassionate other, eventually, turned out to be his own grandfather, a man who had been warm in a family of hard men. He had written letters. He had done chair work. He had hit backdraft more than once.

By year five, he was different. His wife told him, at their fortieth anniversary dinner, that she felt like she had married two men. The first one had been the first twenty-five years of their marriage. The second one was the one she was sitting across from now. She was grateful for both. The second one had been a gift she had not expected.

By year ten, the practices had become invisible. He did not think of himself as doing CFT. He just thought of himself as someone who breathed before responding, who spoke to himself with some warmth, who had learned to pause. His blood pressure was lower. He slept better. His relationship with his grown kids had changed. He had become, in his late sixties, a warmer man than he had ever been.

When asked, in a late-life interview with a local paper about a community award he had received, what he thought had made the biggest difference in his life, he said, without hesitation, "I learned to be kind to myself. I did not know how to before. Learning how changed everything else."

What this means for you: This work can still change you in your fifties, your sixties, your seventies. It is never too late. The pace may be slower. The wins may be quieter. But the arc keeps going, as long as you keep showing up. A practice you sustain for thirty years changes more than a practice you master in thirty weeks and then abandon.

20.7 When It Doesn't Work

Some readers, at the end of this book, will feel that the work has not really landed for them. If that is you, here are options.

Go back to the practices that gave you any traction. Not the ones that looked most appealing. The ones that actually produced any shift, even a small one. Double down on those for a few months before trying anything else.

Consider a therapist. Some of the barriers to this work are not book-solvable. A therapist can help you see what you cannot see on your own, and hold what is too big to hold alone.

Consider that the timing may not be right. Some books meet you at the wrong moment. Put this one on the shelf. Come back in a year, or two, or ten. The book will keep. Your nervous system will keep changing in the meantime, with or without this particular practice. When the timing is right, the book will work differently.

Consider that the fit may not be right. Not every approach works for every person. If CFT has not landed, something else might. Internal Family Systems. Somatic Experiencing. Mindful

Self-Compassion. EMDR. ACT. Good therapy in almost any modality. Your path to something better does not have to be this one.

Do not conclude, from the fact that this book did not transform you, that nothing will. Many, many people have struggled with self-criticism for decades before finding something that helped. Your something-that-helps may still be ahead of you.

20.8 Going Forward

You have reached the end of this book. What you do from here is more important than anything you have done so far.

The practices in this book are not a program with a completion date. They are a set of tools you can carry for the rest of your life. You can pick them up when you need them. You can put them down when you do not. You can come back to any of them at any point, and they will still be there.

The compassionate self you have met in these pages is not a new addition to you. It was always part of you. What you have done, by reading this book, is find the door. Walking through the door is something you will do, or not do, many times in the years ahead. Each walking through is a small act of courage. Each return to the critic, after a stretch of compassion, is human. Each return to the compassion, after a stretch of the critic, is growth.

The critic is not going anywhere. It will still show up. It will still speak. Some days it will be loud. Some days it will be right about something. But you have tools now. You have a different voice to speak from. You have ways of pausing, noticing, asking what the critic is afraid of, and choosing a response that does not leave you smaller than when you started.

Your body has learned something new. Slow breath in, slow breath out, long on the exhale. Hand on the chest. Soft face. A kind sentence in a difficult moment. These are small things. They accumulate into a different life, not quickly, but reliably, if you keep coming back.

You do not have to be good at this. You just have to keep coming back. Six months from now, you will have practiced a bit more. A year from now, more still. Five years from now, if you keep going, you will have changed in ways you cannot yet see from here.

Thank you for reading. Keep going.

A Note On Getting Extra Support

This book was built to be useful on its own. Many readers will get real value from the practices without any other help. Many others will not, and their difficulty is not a sign of weakness or of not trying hard enough. Some things are too big for a book. They need a human in the room.

If you are at the end of this book and you are still struggling, or if at any point in your reading you felt the material reaching into something that felt too large to hold alone, please consider the options below. Reaching for support is one of the most self-compassionate things you can do. It is also, in many cases, the move that makes the practices in this book actually work.

When Extra Support Would Help

Consider getting professional help if any of the following fit your situation.

You have a significant trauma history. Childhood abuse or neglect, assault, combat exposure, a major accident, prolonged domestic violence, medical trauma, or sustained early attachment disruption. Trauma material is often outside the range of what a book can hold safely. A trauma-informed therapist will help you make faster, safer progress than solo work alone.

You have a mental health condition that is not well managed. Depression, anxiety, PTSD, eating disorders, substance use concerns, bipolar conditions, and others. The practices in this book can complement treatment, not replace it. A clinician can help you use the tools in a way that fits your overall plan.

You are experiencing thoughts of harming yourself, thoughts of suicide, or intense hopelessness. Please reach out for professional help right away. The support resources later in this section can help you find a starting point.

The practices keep activating something too large for you to move through. Backdraft that will not settle. Flashbacks. Dissociation. Waves of feeling that disrupt your functioning for days. These are signals that your system needs more support, not less practice. A therapist can help your nervous system hold what is coming up.

You have been practicing for six months or more and feel genuinely stuck. Not the normal slumps described in Chapter 20, but a deeper sense that something is in the way and you cannot see it. A therapist can often see what you cannot see on your own.

You want to go further than a book can take you. Books are foundations. Therapy is architecture. If you are ready to build more than a foundation, a therapist is the next step.

Finding A CFT Therapist

CFT is a recognized therapy modality with trained practitioners around the world. To find a clinician trained in CFT specifically, search for directories maintained by the Compassionate Mind Foundation, which is the organization founded by Paul Gilbert. They keep a list of practitioners who have completed formal CFT training. Many countries also have local CFT networks with their own directories. Searching for "compassion focused therapy practitioner" followed by your region will usually find them.

If a CFT-specific therapist is not available near you (which is common in many regions), a therapist trained in any of the following traditions can work well with the material in this book: compassion-focused therapy, mindful self-compassion, internal family systems, emotion-focused therapy, schema therapy, acceptance and commitment therapy, or general cognitive-behavioral therapy with a warm, relational style. Ask a prospective therapist, directly, if they work with self-criticism, shame, or the inner critic. The answer will tell you a lot.

If cost is an issue, look for sliding-scale clinics, university training clinics (where supervised graduate students offer therapy at reduced rates), community mental health centers, and employee assistance programs through your workplace. Some online therapy platforms also offer reduced pricing. Insurance coverage varies significantly; a call to your insurer to ask about mental health benefits is usually worth the time.

General Therapy Finder Resources

If you are starting from scratch, the following kinds of directories can help you find a therapist. These exist in most countries; the specific names vary.

In the United States, the Psychology Today therapist finder, the American Psychological Association's locator, and SAMHSA's treatment locator are all established starting points. Many states also have licensing-board directories of credentialed providers.

In the United Kingdom, the British Association for Counselling and Psychotherapy (BACP), the British Psychological Society (BPS), and the UK Council for Psychotherapy (UKCP) maintain practitioner directories. The NHS also offers access to Improving Access to Psychological Therapies (IAPT) services.

In Australia, the Australian Psychological Society, the Australian Counselling Association, and Psychology Today Australia have practitioner directories. Medicare rebates for psychological services are available through a GP's Mental Health Treatment Plan.

In Canada, the Canadian Psychological Association and the provincial colleges of psychologists maintain directories. Many employer benefit plans include coverage for psychological services.

If you are in another country, a search for "psychologist directory" or "psychotherapist register" plus your country name will usually find the main licensing-body listing for your region.

Crisis Resources

If you are in immediate danger, or if you are having thoughts of ending your life and need to speak with someone now, please reach out. The services below exist for exactly this moment, and using them is a reasonable act. You do not have to be certain you are in crisis to call. Many services accept calls from people who are not sure.

In the United States, the 988 Suicide and Crisis Lifeline can be reached by calling or texting 988. The Crisis Text Line is reachable by texting HOME to 741741.

In the United Kingdom, the Samaritans can be reached at 116 123 free of charge, any time of day. Shout is a text-based crisis support service reachable by texting SHOUT to 85258.

In Australia, Lifeline can be reached at 13 11 14 any time of day. Beyond Blue offers support at 1300 22 4636. 13YARN (13 92 76) is a support line for Aboriginal and Torres Strait Islander people.

In Canada, Talk Suicide Canada can be reached at 1-833-456-4566. The Kids Help Phone is available at 1-800-668-6868 for young people.

In Ireland, the Samaritans can be reached at 116 123. Pieta House offers support at 1800 247 247.

For immediate physical danger or medical emergency, call your local emergency number: 911 in the US and Canada, 999 in the UK and Ireland, 000 in Australia, 112 across most of Europe.

The International Association for Suicide Prevention maintains a list of crisis lines for countries not listed here. A search for "suicide prevention hotline" plus your country will usually find the relevant numbers.

Policies, privacy, and what happens after a call vary from service to service and from country to country. If you want to know in advance what a particular service offers, most crisis lines publish information about their practices on their own websites. You can also call and ask before you share anything identifying.

A Final Word

Getting help is not the opposite of doing the work. Getting help is doing the work. The people who get the most out of CFT, over the long run, are usually the ones who combined the practices with other forms of support. A therapist. A supportive group. A trusted friend who could hold the hard parts. Medication, where needed. A doctor managing underlying physical contributors. These things add to the practices. They do not subtract from them.

You do not have to do any of this alone. Whatever shape your support takes, putting it in place is not a step backward. It is the step that lets you keep walking forward.

Quick Reference: The Practices At A Glance

What follows is a short, practical summary of every practice in this book, in one place. This section is designed to be returned to. When you are struggling and cannot remember which tool applies, open to this page. Find the one that fits. Use it.

Soothing Rhythm Breathing

Covered in Chapter 11.0

Sit upright. Feet on the floor. Soft face. Hands on thighs. Breathe slowly, letting the exhale be a little longer than the inhale. A common rhythm is four counts in, six counts out. Do this for five to ten minutes. The exhale is where the nervous system settles. The posture and soft face amplify the effect. This is the foundation of every other practice in the book; if only one practice sticks, let it be this one.

Use when: any time of day, as a foundation practice. In crisis moments, even thirty seconds of this resets the escalation.

Safe Place Imagery

Covered in Chapter 12.0

Sit and do three minutes of soothing rhythm breathing first. Then bring a place to mind where your body reads safety. It can be real, imagined, a composite, or something entirely made up. Fill it in one sense at a time: what you see, hear, smell, feel on your skin, maybe taste. Stay for as long as is useful. Return slowly, noticing three things in your actual room before opening your eyes.

Use when: anxiety is high, sleep is hard, a hard moment has passed and you need to settle, or you want to build capacity for the later practices.

The Compassionate Other

Covered in Chapter 13.0

Settle into your safe place using the practice above. Then invite a figure who embodies wisdom, strength, warmth, and caring commitment. The figure can be human, animal, a being of light, a tree, a mountain, or anything your body reads as fully on your side. Let the figure look at you. Feel their presence. Speak to them silently if you want. Let them receive whatever you need to share. Stay in their company for as long as is useful.

Use when: you need to experience care from outside yourself, especially if self-directed compassion is still too hard, or when you are feeling isolated or alone in something difficult.

The Compassionate Self

Covered in Chapter 10.0

Sit upright, soft face, slow breath. Imagine yourself taking on the role of a deeply compassionate person. Embody four qualities: wisdom (life is hard and suffering is human), strength (you do not collapse in the face of pain), warmth (you genuinely care), and caring commitment (you take wise action on behalf of those you care for). From this posture, turn toward a version of yourself who is struggling and offer presence, not solutions.

Use when: the inner critic has been loud, you have just come through something hard, or you want to deliberately strengthen the inward flow of compassion.

Compassionate Letter Writing

Covered in Chapter 14.0

Paper, pen, fifteen to thirty minutes. Write to yourself as a warm, wise friend would. Start with "Dear [your name]." Acknowledge what has been hard. Validate the feelings. Name what you have endured or accomplished. Offer gentle perspective, not lecturing. Close with presence. Sign it. Keep the letter. Read old letters when you are struggling. Aim for weekly, minimum.

Use when: processing a hard week, working through something that feels stuck, preparing for a difficult event, or marking a transition.

Chair Dialogue With The Critic

Covered in Chapter 15.0

Two chairs facing each other, or one chair and a cushion. Sit in the critic chair and let the critic speak, out loud if you can. Move to the compassionate self chair. Ask the critic what it is actually afraid of. Move back. Let the critic answer. Keep moving between chairs. The critic's real fear is almost always two or three layers beneath the surface attack. Respond from the compassionate self with acknowledgment, not argument.

Use when: the critic has been running hard and arguing with it has not worked, or you want to understand a recurring self-attack more deeply. Best done at home with time to settle afterward.

The Self-Compassion Break

Covered in Chapter 18.0

Thirty seconds. Three steps. First, name what is happening: "This is a hard moment." Second, recognize it is part of being human: "Other people feel this too." Third, offer yourself kindness: "May I give myself what I need right now." Hand on chest optional. Silent or aloud. Works anywhere.

Use when: the middle of a stressful day, before a hard conversation, after a hard conversation, in the car, in the bathroom, in a meeting, at a red light.

The Pause

Covered in Chapter 19.0

Two to three seconds between someone else's action and your response. During the pause: one slow breath and one silent question to yourself: "What am I actually feeling?" Then respond. The response that comes after a pause is almost always different from the one that would have come without it.

Use when: you are about to react to someone and want to choose the response rather than react out of the threat system. The single most useful relational skill from the whole book.

Micro-Anchors

Covered in Chapter 18.0

Attach a micro-practice to something you were already doing. Walking through a doorway (one breath). Red lights (one slow-breath cycle). Turning on a faucet (one breath before). Phone notifications (one breath before looking). Before meals (hand on belly, one breath). Bedtime (one kind sentence about the day). Pick one. Build it for two weeks before adding another.

Use when: you want the practice to live in your daily life rather than in a separate block of time. Micro-anchors, over months, produce more change than occasional formal sessions.

The Three Flows Check

Covered in Chapter 9.0

Diagnostic, not a practice. Ask yourself three questions. First, how easily can you feel compassion for a struggling friend? Second, when someone offers you care, how easily do you let it land? Third, when you fail, how do you speak to yourself? Most readers find the outward flow is easiest, the incoming flow is uncomfortable, and the inward flow is hardest. Knowing your pattern tells you which practices to prioritize.

Use when: you want to understand where you are stuck or which practices are most likely to move you.

Working With Backdraft

Covered in Chapter 16.0

If a practice brings up a wave of grief, rage, or other intense feeling, do not fight it. Let the wave move. Stop the deep practice. Ground physically: a cold glass of water, a hand on the chest, a weighted blanket. Take a short walk once the peak has passed. Do not practice again immediately; give the system a day or two. Return to the simpler practices first. Write about what came up once you are settled.

Use when: old material has surfaced and needs to be held, not pushed away.

Trauma-Sensitive Modifications

Covered in Chapter 17.0

If standard practices activate your trauma, adapt them. Keep eyes open, focused on a neutral object. Shorten to one or two minutes. Practice during the day, not at night. Hold something warm. Choose a safe place that is small and contained. Choose a non-human compassionate other (animal, tree, mountain, being of light). Work with a trauma-informed therapist for the deeper practices.

Use when: your history makes the standard versions of the practices activating rather than settling.

Repair After Rupture

Covered in Chapter 19.0

When something has gone wrong in a relationship: acknowledge specifically what you did (not "I am sorry for what happened" but "I am sorry for what I did"). Own your part without over-explaining. Acknowledge the impact on the other person. Commit to something specific going forward. Do not demand forgiveness. Repair is one-sided; you make the repair and the other person decides what to do with it.

Use when: after you have hurt someone and the relationship matters to you. Repair is more important than avoiding rupture; rupture is inevitable, and repair is what keeps relationships healthy.

Quick Map For Common Moments

When you cannot sleep: slow breathing with extended exhale, in bed, until the nervous system settles.

When the critic is loud: name the voice ("the critic is speaking"), ask what it is afraid of, respond from the compassionate self. Or, if the attack is a familiar one, the chair dialogue.

When you are about to react badly: the pause. Two seconds. One breath. One question to yourself.

When you feel ashamed: the self-compassion break, then, if time allows, a letter to yourself.

When you are overwhelmed: safe place imagery, for as long as you have.

When someone you love is struggling: offer presence, not solutions. The same two psychologies (sensitivity and committed action) apply to others as to yourself.

When you have failed at something: notice the critic arriving. Do not argue with it. Write a kind letter to yourself. Or, if time is short, the self-compassion break.

When you are tired: skip the formal practice. Do one micro-practice at one anchor. That is enough.

When you are in crisis: the practices are not a substitute for getting help. Reach out to a therapist, a crisis line, or a trusted person.

Reference

- Beck, A. T., & Haigh, E. A. P. (2014). Advances in cognitive theory and therapy: The generic cognitive model. *Annual Review of Clinical Psychology, 10*, 1–24.

- Beck, J. S. (2021). *Cognitive behavior therapy: Basics and beyond* (3rd ed.). Guilford Press.

- Blatt, S. J. (2004). *Experiences of depression: Theoretical, clinical, and research perspectives.* American Psychological Association.

- Bowlby, J. (1988). *A secure base: Parent-child attachment and healthy human development.* Basic Books.

- Braehler, C., Gumley, A., Harper, J., Wallace, S., Norrie, J., & Gilbert, P. (2013). Exploring change processes in compassion focused therapy in psychosis: Results of a feasibility randomized controlled trial. *British Journal of Clinical Psychology, 52*(2), 199–214.

- Brewin, C. R., Wheatley, J., Patel, T., Fearon, P., Hackmann, A., Wells, A., Fisher, P., & Myers, S. (2009). Imagery rescripting as a brief stand-alone treatment for depressed patients with intrusive memories. *Behaviour Research and Therapy, 47*(7), 569–576.

- Brown, B. (2018). *Dare to lead: Brave work, tough conversations, whole hearts.* Random House.

- Brown, R. P., & Gerbarg, P. L. (2005). Sudarshan kriya yogic breathing in the treatment of stress, anxiety, and depression: Part II: Clinical applications and guidelines. *Journal of Alternative and Complementary Medicine, 11*(4), 711–717.

- Carter, C. S. (1998). Neuroendocrine perspectives on social attachment and love. *Psychoneuroendocrinology, 23*(8), 779–818.

- Cassidy, J., & Shaver, P. R. (Eds.). (2016). *Handbook of attachment: Theory, research, and clinical applications* (3rd ed.). Guilford Press.

- Cosmides, L., & Tooby, J. (2000). Evolutionary psychology and the emotions. In M. Lewis & J. M. Haviland-Jones (Eds.), *Handbook of emotions* (2nd ed., pp. 91–115). Guilford Press.

- Courtois, C. A., & Ford, J. D. (2013). *Treatment of complex trauma: A sequenced, relationship-based approach*. Guilford Press.

- Dearing, R. L., Stuewig, J., & Tangney, J. P. (2005). On the importance of distinguishing shame from guilt: Relations to substance use among female prisoners. *Addictive Behaviors, 30*(7), 1392–1404.

- Depue, R. A., & Morrone-Strupinsky, J. V. (2005). A neurobehavioral model of affiliative bonding: Implications for conceptualizing a human trait of affiliation. *Behavioral and Brain Sciences, 28*(3), 313–350.

- Dickerson, S. S., Gruenewald, T. L., & Kemeny, M. E. (2009). Psychobiological responses to social self-threat: Functional or detrimental? *Self and Identity, 8*(2–3), 270–285.

- Dunne, S., Sheffield, D., & Chilcot, J. (2018). Brief report: Self-compassion, physical health and the mediating role of health-promoting behaviours. *Journal of Health Psychology, 23*(7), 993–999.

- Ehret, A. M., Joormann, J., & Berking, M. (2015). Examining risk and resilience factors for depression: The role of self-compassion and negative self-judgement. *Cognition and Emotion, 29*(8), 1496–1504.

- Eisenberger, N. I. (2012). The pain of social disconnection: Examining the shared neural underpinnings of physical and social pain. *Nature Reviews Neuroscience, 13*(6), 421–434.

- Elliott, R., Watson, J. C., Goldman, R. N., & Greenberg, L. S. (2004). *Learning emotion-focused therapy: The process-experiential approach to change.* American Psychological Association.

- Germer, C. K., & Neff, K. D. (2013). Self-compassion in clinical practice. *Journal of Clinical Psychology, 69*(8), 856–867.

- Germer, C. K., & Neff, K. D. (2015). Cultivating self-compassion in trauma survivors. In V. M. Follette, J. Briere, D. Rozelle, J. W. Hopper, & D. I. Rome (Eds.), *Mindfulness-oriented interventions for trauma: Integrating contemplative practices* (pp. 43–58). Guilford Press.

- Gerritsen, R. J. S., & Band, G. P. H. (2018). Breath of life: The respiratory vagal stimulation model of contemplative activity. *Frontiers in Human Neuroscience, 12*, Article 397.

- Gilbert, P. (2000). The relationship of shame, social anxiety and depression: The role of the evaluation of social rank. *Clinical Psychology & Psychotherapy, 7*(3), 174–189.

- Gilbert, P. (2003). Evolution, social roles, and the differences in shame and guilt. *Social Research, 70*(4), 1205–1230.

- Gilbert, P. (2009). *The compassionate mind: A new approach to life's challenges*. Constable & Robinson.

- Gilbert, P. (2010). *Compassion focused therapy: Distinctive features*. Routledge.

- Gilbert, P. (2014). The origins and nature of compassion focused therapy. *British Journal of Clinical Psychology, 53*(1), 6–41.

- Gilbert, P., & Andrews, B. (Eds.). (1998). *Shame: Interpersonal behavior, psychopathology, and culture*. Oxford University Press.

- Gilbert, P., & Irons, C. (2005). Focused therapies and compassionate mind training for shame and self-attacking. In P. Gilbert (Ed.), *Compassion: Conceptualisations, research and use in psychotherapy* (pp. 263–325). Routledge.

- Gilbert, P., & Procter, S. (2006). Compassionate mind training for people with high shame and self-criticism: Overview and pilot study of a group therapy approach. *Clinical Psychology & Psychotherapy, 13*(6), 353–379.

- Gilbert, P., Clarke, M., Hempel, S., Miles, J. N. V., & Irons, C. (2004). Criticizing and reassuring oneself: An exploration of forms, styles and reasons in female students. *British Journal of Clinical Psychology, 43*(1), 31–50.

- Gilbert, P., McEwan, K., Matos, M., & Rivis, A. (2011). Fears of compassion: Development of three self-report measures. *Psychology and Psychotherapy: Theory, Research and Practice, 84*(3), 239–255.

- Goetz, J. L., Keltner, D., & Simon-Thomas, E. (2010). Compassion: An evolutionary analysis and empirical review. *Psychological Bulletin, 136*(3), 351–374.

- Gottman, J. M., & Silver, N. (2015). *The seven principles for making marriage work*. Harmony Books.

- Greenberg, L. S., Rice, L. N., & Elliott, R. (1993). *Facilitating emotional change: The moment-by-moment process*. Guilford Press.

- Hackmann, A., Bennett-Levy, J., & Holmes, E. A. (2011). *Oxford guide to imagery in cognitive therapy*. Oxford University Press.

- Haidt, J. (2006). *The happiness hypothesis: Finding modern truth in ancient wisdom*. Basic Books.

- Hartig, T., Mitchell, R., de Vries, S., & Frumkin, H. (2014). Nature and health. *Annual Review of Public Health, 35*, 207–228.

- Herman, J. L. (1992). *Trauma and recovery: The aftermath of violence*. Basic Books.

- Holmes, E. A., & Mathews, A. (2010). Mental imagery in emotion and emotional disorders. *Clinical Psychology Review, 30*(3), 349–362.

- Irons, C., & Beaumont, E. (2017). *The compassionate mind workbook: A step-by-step guide to developing your compassionate self*. Robinson.

- Jerath, R., Edry, J. W., Barnes, V. A., & Jerath, V. (2006). Physiology of long pranayamic breathing: Neural respiratory elements may provide a mechanism that explains how slow deep breathing shifts the autonomic nervous system. *Medical Hypotheses, 67*(3), 566–571.

- Kabat-Zinn, J. (1994). *Wherever you go, there you are: Mindfulness meditation in everyday life*. Hyperion.

- Kellogg, S. (2015). *Transformational chairwork: Using psychotherapeutic dialogues in clinical practice*. Rowman & Littlefield.

- Kelly, A. C., Carter, J. C., & Borairi, S. (2014). Are improvements in shame and self-compassion early in eating disorders treatment associated with better patient outcomes? *International Journal of Eating Disorders, 47*(1), 54–64.

- Kim, S., Thibodeau, R., & Jorgensen, R. S. (2011). Shame, guilt, and depressive symptoms: A meta-analytic review. *Psychological Bulletin, 137*(1), 68–96.

- Kirby, J. N. (2017). Compassion interventions: The programmes, the evidence, and implications for research and practice. *Psychology and Psychotherapy: Theory, Research and Practice, 90*(3), 432–455.

- Kirby, J. N., Tellegen, C. L., & Steindl, S. R. (2017). A meta-analysis of compassion-based interventions: Current state of knowledge and future directions. *Behavior Therapy, 48*(6), 778–792.

- Kirschner, H., Kuyken, W., Wright, K., Roberts, H., Brejcha, C., & Karl, A. (2019). Soothing your heart and feeling connected: A new experimental paradigm to study the benefits of self-compassion. *Clinical Psychological Science, 7*(3), 545–565.

- Kok, B. E., Coffey, K. A., Cohn, M. A., Catalino, L. I., Vacharkulksemsuk, T., Algoe, S. B., Brantley, M., & Fredrickson, B. L. (2013). How positive emotions build physical health: Perceived positive social connections account for the upward spiral between positive emotions and vagal tone. *Psychological Science, 24*(7), 1123–1132.

- Kolts, R. L., Bell, T., Bennett-Levy, J., & Irons, C. (2018). *Experiencing compassion-focused therapy from the inside out*. Guilford Press.

- Kreibig, S. D. (2010). Autonomic nervous system activity in emotion: A review. *Biological Psychology, 84*(3), 394–421.

- Laborde, S., Allen, M. S., Borges, U., Dosseville, F., Hosang, T. J., Iskra, M., Mosley, E., Salvotti, C., Spolverato, L., Zammit, N., & Javelle, F. (2022). Effects of voluntary slow breathing on heart rate and heart rate variability. *Neuroscience & Biobehavioral Reviews, 138*, Article 104711.

- Leary, M. R., Tate, E. B., Adams, C. E., Allen, A. B., & Hancock, J. (2007). Self-compassion and reactions to unpleasant self-relevant events. *Journal of Personality and Social Psychology, 92*(5), 887–904.

- Leaviss, J., & Uttley, L. (2015). Psychotherapeutic benefits of compassion-focused therapy: An early systematic review. *Psychological Medicine, 45*(5), 927–945.

- LeDoux, J. E. (1996). *The emotional brain: The mysterious underpinnings of emotional life*. Simon & Schuster.

- Lee, D. A. (2005). The perfect nurturer: A model to develop a compassionate mind within the context of cognitive therapy. In P. Gilbert (Ed.), *Compassion: Conceptualisations, research and use in psychotherapy* (pp. 326–351). Routledge.

- Lieberman, M. D., Eisenberger, N. I., Crockett, M. J., Tom, S. M., Pfeifer, J. H., & Way, B. M. (2007). Putting feelings into words: Affect labeling disrupts amygdala activity in response to affective stimuli. *Psychological Science, 18*(5), 421–428.

- Lutz, A., Brefczynski-Lewis, J., Johnstone, T., & Davidson, R. J. (2008). Regulation of the neural circuitry of emotion by compassion meditation: Effects of meditative expertise. *PLoS ONE, 3*(3), e1897.

- MacBeth, A., & Gumley, A. (2012). Exploring compassion: A meta-analysis of the association between self-compassion and psychopathology. *Clinical Psychology Review, 32*(6), 545–552.

- MacLean, P. D. (1990). *The triune brain in evolution: Role in paleocerebral functions*. Springer.

- Matos, M., & Pinto-Gouveia, J. (2010). Shame as a traumatic memory. *Clinical Psychology & Psychotherapy, 17*(4), 299–312.

- McEwen, B. S. (2007). Physiology and neurobiology of stress and adaptation: Central role of the brain. *Physiological Reviews, 87*(3), 873–904.

- Mikulincer, M., & Shaver, P. R. (2007). *Attachment in adulthood: Structure, dynamics, and change*. Guilford Press.

- Naismith, I., Zarate Guerrero, S., & Feigenbaum, J. (2019). Abuse, invalidation, and lack of early warmth show distinct relationships with self-criticism, self-compassion, and fear of self-compassion. *Clinical Psychology & Psychotherapy, 26*(3), 350–361.

- Neff, K. D. (2003). Self-compassion: An alternative conceptualization of a healthy attitude toward oneself. *Self and Identity, 2*(2), 85–101.

- Neff, K. D. (2011). *Self-compassion: The proven power of being kind to yourself.* William Morrow.

- Neff, K. D., & Beretvas, S. N. (2013). The role of self-compassion in romantic relationships. *Self and Identity, 12*(1), 78–98.

- Neff, K. D., & Germer, C. K. (2013). A pilot study and randomized controlled trial of the mindful self-compassion program. *Journal of Clinical Psychology, 69*(1), 28–44.

- Neff, K. D., & Germer, C. K. (2018). *The mindful self-compassion workbook: A proven way to accept yourself, build inner strength, and thrive.* Guilford Press.

- Neff, K. D., Hsieh, Y.-P., & Dejitterat, K. (2005). Self-compassion, achievement goals, and coping with academic failure. *Self and Identity, 4*(3), 263–287.

- Nesse, R. M. (2019). *Good reasons for bad feelings: Insights from the frontier of evolutionary psychiatry.* Dutton.

- Ogden, P., Minton, K., & Pain, C. (2006). *Trauma and the body: A sensorimotor approach to psychotherapy.* W. W. Norton.

- Öhman, A., & Mineka, S. (2001). Fears, phobias, and preparedness: Toward an evolved module of fear and fear learning. *Psychological Review, 108*(3), 483–522.

- Panksepp, J. (1998). *Affective neuroscience: The foundations of human and animal emotions.* Oxford University Press.

- Pauley, G., & McPherson, S. (2010). The experience and meaning of compassion and self-compassion for individuals with depression or anxiety. *Psychology and Psychotherapy: Theory, Research and Practice, 83*(2), 129–143.

- Pennebaker, J. W. (1997). Writing about emotional experiences as a therapeutic process. *Psychological Science, 8*(3), 162–166.

- Pennebaker, J. W., & Smyth, J. M. (2016). *Opening up by writing it down: How expressive writing improves health and eases emotional pain* (3rd ed.). Guilford Press.

- Porges, S. W. (2007). The polyvagal perspective. *Biological Psychology, 74*(2), 116–143.

- Porges, S. W. (2011). *The polyvagal theory: Neurophysiological foundations of emotions, attachment, communication, and self-regulation.* W. W. Norton.

- Rockliff, H., Karl, A., McEwan, K., Gilbert, J., Matos, M., & Gilbert, P. (2011). Effects of intranasal oxytocin on compassion focused imagery. *Emotion, 11*(6), 1388–1396.

- Russo, M. A., Santarelli, D. M., & O'Rourke, D. (2017). The physiological effects of slow breathing in the healthy human. *Breathe, 13*(4), 298–309.

- Salzberg, S. (1995). *Lovingkindness: The revolutionary art of happiness*. Shambhala.

- Salzberg, S. (2017). *Real love: The art of mindful connection*. Flatiron Books.

- Sapolsky, R. M. (2004). *Why zebras don't get ulcers* (3rd ed.). Holt Paperbacks.

- Schore, A. N. (2012). *The science of the art of psychotherapy*. W. W. Norton.

- Shahar, B., Carlin, E. R., Engle, D. E., Hegde, J., Szepsenwol, O., & Arkowitz, H. (2012). A pilot investigation of emotion-focused two-chair dialogue intervention for self-criticism. *Clinical Psychology & Psychotherapy, 19*(6), 496–507.

- Shahar, G. (2015). *Erosion: The psychopathology of self-criticism*. Oxford University Press.

- Shapira, L. B., & Mongrain, M. (2010). The benefits of self-compassion and optimism exercises for individuals vulnerable to depression. *The Journal of Positive Psychology, 5*(5), 377–389.

- Siegel, D. J. (2012). *The developing mind: How relationships and the brain interact to shape who we are* (2nd ed.). Guilford Press.

- Siegel, D. J., & Hartzell, M. (2003). *Parenting from the inside out*. Jeremy P. Tarcher.

- Singer, T., & Klimecki, O. M. (2014). Empathy and compassion. *Current Biology, 24*(18), R875–R878.

- Sirois, F. M., Kitner, R., & Hirsch, J. K. (2015). Self-compassion, affect, and health-promoting behaviors. *Health Psychology, 34*(6), 661–669.

- Smyth, J. M., Stone, A. A., Hurewitz, A., & Kaell, A. (1999). Effects of writing about stressful experiences on symptom reduction in patients with asthma or rheumatoid arthritis. *JAMA, 281*(14), 1304–1309.

- Steindl, S. R., Kirby, J. N., & Tellegan, C. (2018). Motivational interviewing in compassion-based interventions: Theory and practical applications. *Clinical Psychologist, 22*(3), 265–279.

- Stinckens, N., Lietaer, G., & Leijssen, M. (2013). Working with the inner critic: Therapeutic approach. *Person-Centered & Experiential Psychotherapies, 12*(2), 141–156.

- Tangney, J. P., & Dearing, R. L. (2002). *Shame and guilt*. Guilford Press.

- Tangney, J. P., Stuewig, J., & Mashek, D. J. (2007). Moral emotions and moral behavior. *Annual Review of Psychology, 58*, 345–372.

- Terry, M. L., & Leary, M. R. (2011). Self-compassion, self-regulation, and health. *Self and Identity, 10*(3), 352–362.

- Tsang, J. A., Schulwitz, A., & Carlisle, R. D. (2012). An experimental test of the relationship between self-compassion and forgiveness. *The Journal of Positive Psychology, 7*(6), 486–497.

- Uvnäs-Moberg, K. (1998). Oxytocin may mediate the benefits of positive social interaction and emotions. *Psychoneuroendocrinology, 23*(8), 819–835.

- van der Kolk, B. A. (2014). *The body keeps the score: Brain, mind, and body in the healing of trauma*. Viking.

- Warren, R., Smeets, E., & Neff, K. D. (2016). Self-criticism and self-compassion: Risk and resilience. *Current Psychiatry, 15*(12), 18–21, 24–28, 32.

- Welford, M. (2012). *The compassionate mind approach to building self-confidence*. Robinson.

- Werner, A. M., Tibubos, A. N., Rohrmann, S., & Reiss, N. (2019). The clinical trait self-criticism and its relation to psychopathology: A systematic review. *Journal of Affective Disorders, 246*, 530–547.

- Whelton, W. J., & Greenberg, L. S. (2005). Emotion in self-criticism. *Personality and Individual Differences, 38*(7), 1583–1595.

- Wong, C. C. Y., & Mak, W. W. S. (2013). Differentiating the role of three self-compassion components in buffering cognitive-personality vulnerability to depression. *Journal of Counseling Psychology, 60*(1), 162–169.

- Wood, W., & Neal, D. T. (2007). A new look at habits and the habit-goal interface. *Psychological Review, 114*(4), 843–863.

- Yarnell, L. M., & Neff, K. D. (2013). Self-compassion, interpersonal conflict resolutions, and well-being. *Self and Identity, 12*(2), 146–159.

- Zaccaro, A., Piarulli, A., Laurino, M., Garbella, E., Menicucci, D., Neri, B., & Gemignani, A. (2018). How breath-control can change your life: A systematic review on psycho-physiological correlates of slow breathing. *Frontiers in Human Neuroscience, 12*, Article 353.

- Zessin, U., Dickhäuser, O., & Garbade, S. (2015). The relationship between self-compassion and well-being: A meta-analysis. *Applied Psychology: Health and Well-Being, 7*(3), 340–364.

- Zuroff, D. C., Igreja, I., & Mongrain, M. (1990). Dysfunctional attitudes, dependency, and self-criticism as predictors of depressive mood states. *Personality and Individual Differences, 11*(4), 315–326.

- Zuroff, D. C., Kelly, A. C., Leybman, M. J., Blatt, S. J., & Wampold, B. E. (2010). Between-therapist and within-therapist differences in the quality of the therapeutic relationship: Effects on maladjustment and self-critical perfectionism. *Journal of Clinical Psychology, 66*(7), 681–697.

9 781764 639057